MW01141213

HEALTH SERVICE SUPPORT

The Operational Art:
Canadian Perspectives

Health Service Support

Edited by
Allan English and James C. Taylor

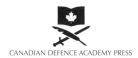

CANADIAN DEFENCE ACADEMY PRESS

Canadian Defence Academy Press
PO Box 17000 Stn Forces
Kingston, Ontario   K7K 7B4

Produced for the Canadian Defence Academy Press
by 17 Wing Winnipeg Publishing Office.
WPO30215

Cover Photo: Courtesy of Dr. Anne Irwin, University of Calgary

Library and Archives Canada Cataloguing in Publication

The operational art : Canadian perspectives : health service support /
edited by Allan English and James C. Taylor.

Issued by Canadian Defence Academy.
Includes bibliographical references.
ISBN 0-662-44240-7 (bound) -- ISBN 0-662-44241-5 (pbk.)
Cat. no.: D4-3/3-1-2007E (bound) -- Cat. no.: D4-3/3-2-2007E (pbk.)

1. Canada--Armed Forces--Medical care. 2. Canada--Armed Forces--
Sanitary affairs. 3. Medicine, Military--Canada. 4. Canada--Armed Forces--
Transport of sick and wounded. I. English, Allan D. (Allan Douglas), 1949-
II. Taylor, James C III. Canadian Defence Academy IV. Title: Health services
support.

UA600.O63 2006   355.3'450971   C2006-980290-4

Printed in Canada.
1 3 5 7 9 10 8 6 4 2

TABLE OF CONTENTS

FOREWORD

I am pleased to commend to you this volume, the third in the Canadian Defence Academy's series on the Operational Art. It reflects Canada's participation in the ongoing discussion amongst North Atlantic Treaty Organization nations regarding the evolution of Health Service Support (HSS) in the modern security environment. Its inclusion within this important series of publications promotes an increasing awareness by the Canadian Forces (CF) of the integral nature of HSS in operational planning, and a better appreciation by operational commanders of the doctrine and roles of their HSS elements.

This volume comprises the combined works of a number of our Canadian Forces Health Services (CFHS) leaders, produced in the course of their military education; it comes at a particularly opportune time as our organization is in the process of transformation. The CFHS is currently implementing an ambitious and innovative health care reform process, the goal of which is to develop a patient-oriented health service that enhances operational effectiveness and better meets the needs of our soldiers, sailors and air personnel, both at home and abroad. This book is reflective of that fundamental evolution, and I am confident that it will be a valuable contribution to the ongoing dialogue of the profession of arms in Canada.

MILITI SUCCURIMUS / SANITAS IN ORE

Margaret F. Kavanagh
Commodore
Commander, Canadian Forces Health Services Group

INTRODUCTION

Allan English and Colonel James C. Taylor

This volume, *The Operational Art: Canadian Perspectives – Health Service Support*, is the third in a series published by the Canadian Defence Academy Press. It follows *The Operational Art: Canadian Perspectives – Context and Concepts* (2005) and *The Operational Art: Canadian Perspectives – Leadership and Command* (2006). The purpose of these volumes is to offer perspectives on distinct Canadian approaches to the operational art, based on our national and military cultures and historical experience.

A growing body of work is addressing how Health Service Support (HSS) can be transformed to meet the challenges of current and future security environments, and this book aims to contribute to this literature.[1] Commissioned by the Commander Canadian Forces Health Services Group, this volume articulates the nature of health service support, depicts and interprets various concepts of health service support, and examines HSS doctrinal concepts in a Canadian context at the operational level. It is based on the writings of HSS senior officers on issues related to HSS done while conducting professional military education at the Canadian Forces College (CFC) and postgraduate education at Royal Roads University. This volume showcases these works so that they are available for the use of military professionals and others who are facing new challenges in the study and practice of the operational art.

The roots of this project are, however, deeper than those described in the preceding paragraph. One might ask for example, how did Canadian HSS professionals come to write about HSS and the operational art? One answer to this question can be found in the origins of the Advanced Military Studies Course (AMSC), which was designed to focus on "the study of war and operations other than war at the operational level with additional emphasis on intellectual and professional development in related areas."[2] The first AMSC (September to November 1998) treated all support functions as peripheral to the operational art, a view that was not uncommon at the time among Canadian senior officers. There was a great deal of resistance at CFC to straying from what was seen to be the proper path for AMSC studies. This path was created based on the assumption that since the operational art was clearly about "operations" and the course was primarily for "operators," the subject matter should focus on "operations," and support issues should be tangential to the course.

After the first AMSC, however, based on Jack English's observation that operational art was characterized by staggering logistics and staff planning as much as by sweeping battlefield manoeuvre,[3] those involved in AMSC curriculum development realized that support factors deserved more attention in the studies on the course. Therefore, beginning with AMSC 2 (September to December 1999), new portions related to logistics and personnel support were added to the curriculum. On AMSC 2, the term "sustainment" was used by Allan English to signify the co-ordination of all support at the operational level. In this context, the use of the term "sustainment" created some controversy because it did not correspond to what some envisioned sustainment to be, as depicted in more limited definitions of the term.[4] Nevertheless, for lack of a better term, it was used on AMSC to try to raise the level of debate from primarily technical and stovepiped approaches to logistics and personnel policies to approaches based on a holistic study of support functions. Using this holistic approach, some AMSC student research papers found that there were flaws in Canadian and Allied support doctrine and structures, largely because support issues were dealt with in isolation, and that these flaws had a serious negative impact on the ability of the CF and Allied forces to conduct campaigns.[5] A combination of these papers and literature reviews convinced most AMSC students and staff that existing doctrine did not adequately take into account the integrated nature of the materiel and human resource aspects of campaign planning and execution. It was also found that, while the materiel aspects of theatre-level sustainment were relatively well addressed by logistics doctrine, the doctrine relating to the human resource aspects of campaign planning and execution was fragmented and very general in nature. An important initiative in this approach to studying sustainment, therefore, was the holistic examination of sustainment as a complex, linked system, recognizing that actions in one part of the system had effects on other parts of the system. Beginning in 1999, key concepts and principles of the human dimension of sustainment were examined by some at CFC in an attempt to stimulate debate about new concepts and doctrine on this subject, with an emphasis on support to joint and combined operations, integrating approaches to personnel and material support, health services support policies, and the human dimension of sustainment, in a Canadian context.

At the beginning of the 21st century, Western militaries are struggling to develop sustainment systems to cope with a variety of dispersed, non-contiguous, joint and other types of operations simultaneously. In this new security environment, some have observed that "deployment, employment and sustainment are beginning to merge."[6] The addition of concepts like "Joint, Interagency, Multinational, and Public" (JIMP), "3D" (defence, diplomacy and development), and "integrated" to the national security lexicon at the beginning of the 21st century will no doubt also impact military sustainment. For example, in "integrated" operations, military sustainment may take on new dimensions as it goes beyond its traditional boundaries in the requirement to support "integrated" teams. The new security environment has also caused some to observe that the traditional levels of war are beginning to merge, to be compressed, or to be blurred. Others have noted that even if the traditional levels still exist, it is not productive to over-compartmentalize operations into what could be termed artificial levels like strategic, operational and tactical.[7] All of these factors contribute to making the holistic study of sustainment at the operational level a complex undertaking. However, it is an undertaking that cannot be avoided if we are to face the challenges of the new security environment successfully, because, as recently as Operation Apollo (2001-2003),[8] it was noted that sustainment considerations have been "an afterthought in the operational planning process."[9]

Another controversy related to the human dimension of support, besides the place that support should take in the curriculum of a course focusing on the operational art, had come to a head at CFC by AMSC 5, in 2002, when, given the presumed "operator" focus of AMSC, some challenged the decision to include HSS officers on the course.

While one would not expect HSS personnel to command combat formations in today's increasingly complex security environment, it is realistic, based on CF doctrine, to expect that HSS personnel, as military professionals, should be able to contribute effectively to the planning and execution of a campaign. The roles that HSS personnel will play in 21st century operations will demand of them a wider range of competencies, outside of their traditional specialties, than has been the case in the past.

Duty with Honour: The Profession of Arms in Canada, "a defining document for Canada's profession of arms" and a "cornerstone document" for the CF,[10] describes the philosophy and practice of the profession of arms in Canada, and gives guidance on how HSS professionals fit into the profession of arms in this country. This document describes the Canadian military profession as "a collective profession" because "no individual or even a subgroup of individuals can accomplish" the roles and missions of the CF. *Duty with Honour* also notes that "[a] higher degree of organization and specialization is therefore required for collective professions than is normal for associational professions."[11] Furthermore, it recognizes that the military profession in Canada includes individuals, such as HSS personnel, who are also members of civilian professions. According to *Duty with Honour*, such "dual professionals," as well as mastering their civilian professions, must accept the duties and responsibilities of membership in the profession of arms. Among other things, this includes mastering what it calls the "common body of knowledge" of the profession of arms in Canada. *Duty with Honour* goes on to say that specialists in uniform are "first and foremost" members of the profession of arms, and that they are, therefore, required "to have a basic understanding of the generation and use of armed force" that allows them to relate their work to the goals and missions of the CF.[12] We would argue, therefore, that for the CF to be effective in the new security environment, a selected cohort of HSS personnel must acquire expertise in certain aspects of the operational art. This implies that some HSS personnel need not only technical competency in their health profession, but also highly developed competencies in some aspects of the operational art and, perhaps thereafter, the strategic art.

The first two chapters in this volume set the stage for what follows by providing an overview of how ongoing changes in military operations and operational concepts pose major challenges to military health care support that in some ways continue to rely on Cold War models. In the first chapter, Salisbury and English note that 21st century operations will be conducted in a more diffuse batttlespace, thereby producing different and somewhat unpredictable rates and types of casualties than experienced in the past. These operations pose challenges in developing a medical support plan, as current concepts based on a concentration of effort and tiered support may not be the most effective means of providing timely care. Moreover, technological solutions in medicine to these challenges, in addition to providing for a more robust response, will also pose ethical and legal challenges to military medicine. They conclude that if Canada wishes to put its military personnel in harm's way, then it must adopt a new approach to medical support if it is to be prepared to sustain them with appropriate Canadian military health care support. In the second chapter, Bernier examines threats to operational force health protection. He reminds us that that in most military operations the majority of casualties (and often deaths) have resulted from disease and non-battle injuries (DNBI) rather than from hostile action. Despite advances in modern medicine, DNBI casualties have continued to adversely affect CF operations and those of our major allies in recent years, and yet most are unnecessary and preventable. He concludes that command efforts to protect deployed CF elements are being complicated by a number of factors, including inadequate command awareness of and attention to health protection issues, and the late or inadequate consideration of medical input to the planning process. Bernier argues that, in order to minimize preventable DNBI casualties, health protection issues should be an important part of all levels of command and staff training.

The next four chapters debate how Canadian military health care support can best be provided from an operational-level perspective. In the third chapter, Taylor addresses the requirements for a deployable HSS capability that is valid across all CF force planning scenarios, that is benchmarked to a Canadian civilian level of care, and that is interoperable with our principal allies. He argues that the widely used "hub-and-spoke" HSS model, whereby patients are aeromedically evacuated from point of injury directly to a Role 3 HSS facility, has numerous limitations. Therefore, he concludes that an effective HSS system on the modern conventional battlefield will still require a robust forward surgical and evacuation capability. Furthermore, he contends that, for land casualty management, these requirements can be met by an evolved Role 2+ CF Field Ambulance, making it a key capability in the patient care continuum across the spectrum of conflict. In the fourth chapter Weger builds on Taylor's argument that the CF requires a robust forward surgical and evacuation based on an evolved CF Field Ambulance. Weger argues that the CF requires lightweight, very mobile HSS elements that can operate as close to the fighting as the tactical situation allows and thereby provide resuscitative surgery to stabilize casualties for further evacuation. However, he notes that current CF HSS doctrine will need to be modified to redefine Role 2 operational HSS to include initial resuscitative surgery and to support this redefinition with the establishment of a Far Forward Surgical capability integral to Canadian field ambulances if HSS is to be able to adequately support CF units in the future battlespace. In the fifth chapter, Mitchell expands on these concepts by analyzing recent American and British operations, and she maintains that the field ambulance organizations as they currently exist in the CF have limited utility in modern operations. She asserts that the realities of the emerging battlespace will force medical planners to balance mobility and definitive treatment, the location of surgical capabilities and the proper skill set of medical personnel in support of future operations. And she concludes that, in order to meet the challenges of the future battlespace, CF HSS needs to restructure existing field ambulance organizations along the lines of modular, building block capabilities. In the sixth chapter, Molyneaux addresses dental aspects of HSS in the future battlespace. He argues, similar to Mitchell, that dental health services support to operations must be organized around a basic and common "building block" section capable of providing clinical dental treatment, either independently or with other modules, and that this capability module must be readily deployable, modern, and interoperable with our allies. Molyneaux notes that changes in equipment, organization and doctrine will be required to effect these changes.

The final two chapters of this book examine issues that relate to the future of HSS. In the penultimate chapter, Patterson uses the Canadian Navy's Joint Support Ship (JSS), a multipurpose ship that will provide surge sealift, underway replenishment, support to forces ashore, and a level of medical coverage that exceeds anything currently provided by the Canadian Navy, as a case study in the effects of HSS considerations on operational planning. She concludes that the multi-layering of tasks on the JSS may result in the inability to commit to two or more major tasks without degrading support to other tasks. Furthermore, she asserts that the lack of comprehensive CF joint doctrine compounds the challenge of realizing the full extent of the JSS supporting capabilities as various JSS functions compete for primacy without authoritative doctrinal guidance. In the last chapter, Taylor argues that CFHS strategic leader development must be transformed to ensure that the CFHS has a sustainable strategic leadership capacity to ensure its success in providing effective HSS in the new security environment. The future strategic leadership of the CFHS will need to ensure that recent changes in CFHS structure, culture and roles evolve appropriately to deal with these future challenges. Therefore, Taylor proposes a CFHS Leader Development Framework to guide the transformation of CFHS strategic leader development. This Framework addresses the "dual competencies," comprising both general CF knowledge and HS professional knowledge, required of CFHS officers as "dual professionals." While Taylor acknowledges that there are substantial costs to developing a sustainable strategic leadership capacity for the CFHS, he contends that this cost is exceeded only by the cost of not developing this capacity to meet the needs of the CF.

The previous book in this series, on leadership and command and the operational art, noted that the evolution of CF joint command and control structures has been ad hoc and often rushed. It also revealed that in the post-Cold War period the CF lacked an effective method of collecting and disseminating lessons learned from various CF operations and that CF joint doctrine was inadequate. These same problems affected sustainment initiatives and doctrine in the CF during that era. The CF has initiated a number of important changes to address these issues, including the creation of Canadian Operational Support Command[13] under recent CF transformation efforts and the ongoing Health Services' transformation, Rx 2000.[14] However, without a proper lessons-learned process to capture and analyze experience and relevant theory, as shown in Figure 1, these initiatives will not develop the required sustainable doctrinal foundation to ensure that they are effective and enduring.

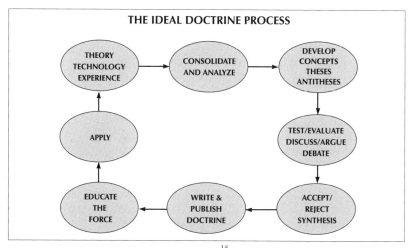

FIGURE 1 - THE IDEAL DOCTRINE PROCESS[15]

If HSS personnel are to make effective contributions to CF transformation, which will ultimately affect how the CF conducts operations in the new security environment, and if HSS personnel are to contribute to the effective planning and execution of campaigns that will animate these operations, selected HSS personnel will need to have a solid grasp of the operational art. In a similar vein, "operators" will need to understand the critical role that HSS plays in the planning and execution of campaigns. With knowledge of how support factors, and HSS in particular, both enable and constrain operational-level activities, HSS personnel and "operators" can function more effectively at the operational level thus enabling more favourable mission outcomes. To achieve the required level of knowledge, theory, experience and doctrine must be captured, debated and disseminated. This book is offered as a contribution to this process.

NOTES

1   This literature is cited in the contributions here. See also Guy S. Strawder, "Transforming Combat Health Support," *Joint Forces Quarterly* Issue 41 (Second Quarter 2006), 60-7.

2   Canadian Forces College (CFC), *Advanced Military Studies Course 2 Syllabus* (Toronto: CFC, May 1999), iii.

3   John English, "The Operational Art: Developments in the Theories of War," in B.J.C. McKercher and Michael A. Hennessy, eds. *The Operational Art: Developments in the Theories of War* (Westport, CT: Praeger, 1996), 19.

4   The official definition of "sustainment" is "The requirement for a military force to maintain its operational capability for the duration required to achieve its objectives. Sustainment consists of the continued supply of consumables, and the replacement of combat losses and non-combat attrition of equipment and personnel. DND, *Canadian Forces Operations*, B-GG-005-004/AF-000, (15 July 2005), p. GL-9, available at http://www.dcds.forces.gc.ca/jointDoc/docs/B-GJ-005-300_e.pdf.

5   See for example Carla Coulson, "Sustaining Joint and Combined Operations: Reflections on the Adequacy   of   Doctrine,"   paper   written   for   AMSC   3,   available   at http://wps.cfc.forces.gc.ca/papers/amsc/amsc3/coulson.htm;   Charles   Davies,   "Sustainment Transformation: If You Don't Know Where You're Going, Any Road Will Get You There," paper written for AMSC 6, available at http://wps.cfc.forces.gc.ca/papers/amsc6/davies.htm; and Bryn M. Weadon, "Canada's Joint Sustainment Co-ordination Capabilities," paper written for AMSC 3, available at http://wps.cfc.forces.gc.ca/papers/amsc/amsc3/weadon.htm.

6   "Exercise   Unified   Quest   2003,   Executive   Report,"   final   draft,   12.   Available   at https://unifiedquest.army.mil/tfw/01_home/Slick_Bks/Slick%20Book%202003.pdf.

7   See for example, Allan English, "The Operational Art," in Allan English et al., eds., *The Operational Art: Canadian Perspectives - Context and Concepts* (Kingston, ON: Canadian Defence Academy Press, 2005), 25-6, 33-4; and Daniel Gosselin, "The Loss of Mission Command for Canadian Expeditionary Operations," in Allan English, ed., *The Operational Art: Canadian Perspectives - Leadership and Command* (Kingston, ON: Canadian Defence Academy Press, 2006), 204-208.

8   "Operation Apollo was Canada's military contribution to the international campaign against terrorism from October 2001 to October 2003." DND, Operations – Past Operations web site – Operation

Apollo, http://www.forces.gc.ca/site/operations/Apollo/index_e.asp

9   Canada, Department of National Defence (DND), DCDS Group, "Operation Apollo – Lessons Learned Staff Action Directive," Annex B to 3350-165/A27, dated April 2003, p. B-39.

10   DND, *Duty with Honour: The Profession of Arms in Canada* (Kingston, ON: CF Leadership Institute, 2003), 1.

11   Ibid., 9. "In an associational profession, members typically function independently, dealing direct-ly with their clients, as is usually the case with the medical and legal professions."

12   Ibid., 51-2.

13   "Canadian Operational Support Command (CANOSCOM) is responsible for providing support to the operational commands including but not limited to logistic, engineering, health services, communi-cations, and military police support, etc." DND, "New Canadian Forces Operational Commands Take Charge of Domestic, Special and International Operations," News Release NR–06.002 (31 January 2006). Available at http://www.forces.gc.ca/site/newsroom/view_news_e.asp?id=1851.

14   "The goal of Rx2000 is to develop and implement solutions for reported health care deficiencies thereby improving the standard of health care provided to CF members at home and abroad," DSP Project 00000297, Section 2.1, dated 19 October 2000. See also DND, *Project Rx2000: An Update* (Canadian Forces Health Services: Ottawa, 2002).

15   From Dennis M. Drew, "Inventing a Doctrine Process," *Airpower Journal* 9, no. 4 (Winter 1995), 42–52.

CHAPTER 1

PROGNOSIS 2020: A MILITARY MEDICAL STRATEGY FOR THE CANADIAN FORCES*

By Colonel (retired) David Salisbury and Allan English

The next twenty years will see major changes in military operational doctrine and tactics, some of which have already been foreshadowed in the ongoing "war on terror."[1] To address these changes, the Canadian Forces' (CF) blueprint for the future, *Strategy 2020*, tells us that the CF intends "to position the force structure of the CF to provide Canada with modern, task-tailored, and globally deployable combat-capable forces that can respond quickly to crises at home and abroad, in joint or combined operations." These goals will have profound effects on the provision of military health support to the CF. The changing nature of the battlefield will not only change the type and number of casualties, it will also change their dispersion on the battlefield. Traditional methods of providing medical support on the battlefield will no longer be the most efficient and effective way of providing trauma care. Therefore, to realize the vision of *Strategy 2020*, a strategy for dealing with the medical issues of sustaining troops on the battlefield of the future must be formulated.

The purpose of this paper is to examine the issues that will affect the formulation of a military medical strategy by looking forward at future trends in military operations and other factors that will affect the CF Health Services. Factors such as the trends in civilian health care that will impact military medicine, changes in military operations brought about by the Revolution in Military Affairs (RMA) and technological changes in providing health care will be examined for their implications for the CF Health Services of 2020. The paper concludes that, in the future, the current concentration of effort and tiered support may not be the most effective means of providing timely care for CF personnel. Advancements in medical care will not only provide a more robust response to battlefield

---

*   This chapter first appeared as David Salisbury and Allan English, "Prognosis 2020: A Military Medical Strategy for the Canadian Forces," *Canadian Military Journal* 4, no.2 (Summer 2003), 45-54.

casualties, but they will also pose ethical and legal challenges to military medicine. The CF's senior leadership will need to understand these issues in order for them to develop optimal logistical support plans for the CF of 2020.

In the past, casualties from disease more often decided the outcome of campaigns than operational art. It is only within the last 100 years that military medicine has significantly reduced the number of deaths and injuries among military forces. In the First World War, the Canadian Expeditionary Force suffered the following fatal casualties: 39,488 killed in action and 12,048 died of wounds. But it was a "medical miracle" that 154,361 survived their wounds and that four out of five soldiers returned to active service. The miracle was that in the First World War, for the first time in a major war, death by enemy action took a heavier toll than disease.[2] Yet the threat of defeat by disease has been a constant companion to modern commanders. For example, it could be argued that Rommel, often considered to be the master of the operational art, defeated himself in North Africa by his inattention to the health of his forces. For every German soldier lost to battle injury in that theatre of operations, three were lost to disease (a return to pre-First World War loss rates). Overall, Rommel lost a force equal to twice his average strength temporarily or permanently to disease, and German soldiers were almost three times as likely to become ineffective for health reasons as their British opponents. Rommel himself was evacuated twice to Germany because of hepatitis. On the other hand, General Sir William Slim under-stood that the health of troops was a commander's responsibility. When he took over 14th Army in Burma in late 1943, the malaria rate was 84 percent per annum of total strength of army. Slim aggressively tackled medical discipline. He believed that more than half the battle against disease was fought by regimental officers not doctors, and he fired regimental officers who did not ensure that malaria prophylaxis measures were taken. As a result of Slim's actions his Army's disease attrition rate dropped from 360 per 1,000 men per month in 1943 to 30 per 1,000 in 1945.[3] More recently, during the Soviet-Afghan War, the Soviet 40th Army paid a price for its poor hygiene practices. Of the 620,000 Soviet troops who served in Afghanistan, 67 percent required hospitalization for a serious illness. At one point, between October and December 1981, the entire 5th Motorized Rifle Division was combat ineffective when more than 3,000 of its men were simultaneously stricken with hepatitis.[4] The recent experience of coalition forces on operations in Afghanistan confirms that these health issues are still vital to maintaining force effectiveness. The loss of a significant cadre of men in the UK International Stabilization Force Afghanistan (ISAF) contingent due to a common viral illness demonstrates that even a well-prepared, well-immunized army can still be done in by the bugs!

The CF Health Services are charged with the responsibility of maintaining the health of Canada's military on operations. It has been referred to as Canada's 14th Health Care System, employing close to 4,500 Regular and Reserve Force personnel as well as over 600 civilians with an annual expenditure of close to $200 million.[5] It is currently undergoing major reform in response to a number of reports and studies that found deficiencies in the care provided to CF members.[6] Although many of these reforms have focused on a future force structure, the predominant focus has been on fixing current and past deficiencies. The notable exception has been the work of the Standing Committee on Operational Medicine Review (SCOMR) that has looked at what the future CF Health Services should do.[7] SCOMR has also tried to identify current capability and technology gaps, and it has suggested a way ahead at the tactical and operational level. However, the CF still has not articulated a comprehensive military medical strategy.

One of the first questions one might ask in formulating such a strategy is why have a military health system at all? A substantial military medical capability sends four important messages to Canadians. First, it tells the people of this country that their leaders have prepared the appropriate means to care for the sons and daughters sent into harm's way. Second, it tells the world that the force is a credible and sustainable fighting force. Third, it tells commanders that they will be supported and sustained. Finally, and perhaps most importantly, it tells the troops that we as a nation care about them. For "in the absence of medical readiness we can have no assurance that our troops, the flesh-and-blood elements of our weapon systems, will retain the will to fight, which is the crucial factor in the equation for victory."[8]

While the foregoing argues that adequate medical care must be provided for all military organizations, it does not present a cogent argument that the care should be provided by a military health care system. To do that one must ask – are there any unique characteristics to military medicine that make it different than civilian medicine practised for military members? A leading American commentator, Captain Arthur Smith, a US Navy physician, contends that there are unique aspects to the practice of military medicine that can be illustrated with two examples. First, the treatment of wounds on the battlefield must be different from the treatment of similar types of wounds found in civilian care. If battlefield wounds are immediately closed, there is a substantial risk of gas gangrene. This is quite different from civilian care where primary closure is the standard procedure. Second, in civilian health care, the assignment of resources is usually done on the basis of greatest individual need because, except in the most exceptional cases, all patients will receive adequate care eventually. In military medicine and some civilian mass casualty situations, the most needy patients must at times be sacrificed in order to save the maximum number of wounded. As Smith says: "To do more than is necessary to stabilize patients and preserve life and limb (if the latter is even possible in the rush of large numbers of casualties) might well effect the lives of many other subsequent patients."[9]

Therefore, most nations accept that a military medical health care system is a necessity.[10] However, some of the models of military health care projected by other countries are inappropriate for Canada. In the case of the US, the size, magnitude and responsibilities of its medical health care system are quite different from ours. The CF Health Services, unlike their US counterparts, are only responsible for care to uniformed personnel. Although Canada can, therefore, concentrate its military medical resources on purely military medical needs, the CF still depends on the Canadian civilian health care system to provide for other needs, such as some aspects of in-garrison primary care, specialist support and the reception of casualties from overseas operations. Thus the state of civilian health care in Canada will have a major impact on the full provision of health care to the CF.

CIVILIAN HEALTH CARE TRENDS

The civilian health care system in Canada is widely considered to be in crisis. In 2001, the Government of Canada established a Royal Commission on the future of health care, popularly known as the Romanow Commission. This commission examined this crisis, developed a dialogue with Canadians on their health care system, and made recommendations to the federal government on a way ahead to address the health care crisis. The Commission also addressed Canadian values and how they are and should be reflected in the *Canada Health Act*. In its final report, published in November 2002, the Commission focused on issues such as sustainability, funding, maintenance of quality, and access to health care as well as issues of leadership, collaboration, and responsibility in the Canadian health care system.[11] All of these issues are of intense interest and import to the CF health care system as changes in any of these dimensions will shape the milieu in which military medicine in Canada operates.

Of the many challenges facing health care in Canada, perhaps the most serious are funding, demographics (the aging population) and the shortage of health care personnel. Furthermore, like the US, there are rising expectations of what health care can and should do for people. Technological changes in informatics, diagnostic imaging and the ongoing biotechnology revolution are profoundly changing the nature of healthcare delivery and driving up costs.

The CF Health Services have not been immune to these challenges, and they, along with others, have been raised in a number of government reports.[12] The CF has also embarked on a major project called Rx2000 to reform the CF Health Services.[13] Rx2000 will not be addressed here directly as its reforms are in response to current and past conditions. Nevertheless, these reforms will shape the ability of the CF Health Services to respond to future operational changes and demands, and they must be implemented with an eye to the future, a future in which the needs for military health care will be quite different from today.

Any debate on health care in Canada, including one on military health care, must address the five principles of Medicare enunciated in the *Canada Health Act*: the need for *Public Administration*, *Comprehensiveness* of care, *Universality* of coverage, *Portability* of coverage and *Accessibility* to necessary physician and hospital services.[14]

The *Canada Health Act* specifically excludes CF members from coverage under the various provincial Medicare plans. However CF members, quite rightly, expect that they will receive the same care and entitlements that all other Canadians receive. Military health care is of course publicly administered, and issues of comprehensiveness are addressed in the spectrum of care offered to CF members that is comparable to provincial plans.[15] Universality is provided to all Regular Force members but is at times problematic for members of the Reserve Force who are only covered by the CF medical system while on certain classes of service. Portability is generally not a problem in Canada for military care, although accessibility often is problematic. While the provision of all these services in Canada is no less a challenge to the military health care system than to the civilian health care system, providing the same level and spectrum of care in the many and varied places the CF is deployed around the world is a daunting task. Like the US, health care in Canada is shifting from an emphasis on hospital based "sick" care to a primary care, prevention-based model with an increasing emphasis on patient (or client) responsibility.[16] This shift in emphasis will profoundly affect military medicine. There is, however, a potential danger that these wider societal changes and the necessary focus of military health care practitioners on meeting civilian norms will erode important military medicine concepts that will result in "the practice of medicine in the military rather than military medicine."[17] For example, civilian care is patient-centric while of necessity, especially in times of war, military medicine must focus on what is the best for the majority.

Perhaps no single change in civilian health care is more important than the changes in the professions that provide care. The two largest regulated professions, nurses and physicians, are re-defining their roles in the system. Nurses are taking on primary care roles previously the sole domain of the doctors, and para-professionals are playing increasing roles in the delivery of care. Physicians, on the other hand, are tending towards more specialization and there is a shortage of family physicians in Canada.[18] The CF is currently experiencing an extreme shortage of medical officers. While this may be ameliorated by current initiatives, the long-term picture for physician availability in Canada points to continuing challenges in this area. Innovative use of the Reserves, civilian health care providers in-garrison, and physician extenders such as nurse practitioners and independent duty medics will help. In the long-term, though, it appears that the mix of providers will have to change. Due to operational necessity, the CF Health Services may have to lead this change, rather than follow civilian practice.

Beaty has emphasized the need for and future of "brilliant medics" on the modern battlefield. He points out that the dispersal of combatants, the scarcity of physicians and surgeons, and the need for rapid stabilization and transport of casualties will necessitate a fundamental change in the way care is delivered on the battlefield of the future.[19] The increasing use of Special Forces, where the protections of the Geneva Conventions for medical personnel may be ambiguous or irrelevant,[20] will probably dictate the development of the combat medic within the CF. That is, a combatant with sufficient medical training to assist and stabilize fellow combatants on the battlefield. This medic will need to have skills in airway management, hemorrhage control, and the establishment of intravenous infusions that will be applied until the casualty can be evacuated to a medical facility. Such a person will need to be able to fight as a primary role and only provide care as a secondary role. This will be an expanded capability well beyond the current first aid and buddy care model. Innovations in communications, individual monitoring capability and telemedicine will extend the reach of medical personnel and provide more expert and rapid care to the point of wounding to assist the combat medic. But any initiative to develop combat medics will face the same difficulties in licensing and training that the CF encountered with Search and Rescue Technicians (SAR Techs). However, the success the CF has enjoyed with the training and certification of SAR Techs demonstrates that such a concept is feasible.[21]

Nevertheless, preparing military medical personnel for the battlefield will continue to be a challenge. A number of authors have emphasized how even the provision of civilian trauma care does not prepare one for the provision of battlefield care.[22] Furthermore, the difficulty in training CF surgeons is even more acute than that of their US confreres as the incidence of gunshot wounds and other penetrating trauma is so much less in Canada than in the US.

The speed of modern combat and the rapidity with which operations will come to an end will not allow enough time for the past methods of learning the lessons of combat surgery on the job in the first few days of combat. This means that surgeons must be trained in peacetime, but as we have seen, the procedures they must master are not appropriate to civilian peacetime trauma medicine.

MILITARY OPERATIONAL TRENDS

In order for the leaders of a military medicine system to devise a strategy for the future, the operational activities and strategic goals of the force as a whole must be understood. *Strategy 2020* and other documents provide some guidance to them, but the strategic visions enunciated in both *Strategy 2020* and the newly released *Army Strategy*[23] have profound implications for the military medical support of the CF. In particular, the move to lighter weight forces that are globally deployable, the "early in, early out" concept, and the increased use of Special Forces with their unique support demands will require innovative and technologically sophisticated medical support solutions.[24]

The RMA has already affected thinking about the future CF, as some believe it will produce "lighter" forces using modern information systems and precision weapons to act rapidly and decisively on the high tech battlefield.[25] While sophisticated technology may enable the use of fewer personnel to achieve the same combat effect, high tech solutions are not necessarily cheaper. A reduced number of very skilled personnel operating these systems means fewer personnel are "at risk" for injury; however, the loss of even one person may have a serious impact on mission outcomes. Therefore, commanders need to be wary of how light the medical support footprint can become, as the RMA may increase the need for highly efficient and effective personnel support functions such as health care. As Smith warns: "To meet the modern mandate for compactness and simplicity in maneuver units, unrealistic medical support expectations have been attached to a warfighting strategy that allows for only minimal medical support function ashore."[26] This is a significant issue for the CF given recent cutbacks and downsizing.

Given the CF's lack of dedicated tactical medical airlift and Canada's overall shortage of strategic airlift, the CF could be entirely dependent on its coalition partners (especially the US) for acceptable military medical care to deployed forces. This reality would dictate a need for not just interoperability but also for commonality in equipment, doctrine and information systems so that CF patients could fit seamlessly into the US health support system. Fortunately, North American health care training standards and practices would make this conceptually easy to achieve; however, lack of independent stand-alone capability would limit the options for employment of the CF without coincident US deployment. But even if coalition partners are prepared to provide necessary medical support to the CF, the more important question is whether Canada is prepared to risk the welfare of its sons and daughters, "placed in harm's way," to the medical coverage and support supplied by another nation.

In the past, this has aroused great passions in this country. During the First World War, the provision of what was perceived to be inadequate medical care by British Volunteer Aid Detachments and, during the Second World War, the treatment of cases of "flying stress" and "lack of morale fibre" in Canadian aircrew by the British military caused such a furore that the Canadian government was forced to intervene.[27] It is ironic that the same governments that had denied adequate resources to the Canadian military to deal with these issues, then demanded immediate solutions in response to the public's insistence that something be done.

The question of the treatment of Canadian military personnel by other nations is exacerbated by the fact that military health systems around the world are experiencing problems with recruiting and re-designing their concept of operations to meet the modern battlefield need.[28] Canada cannot assume that our allies will always provide for us, and the leadership of the CF must be aware of the risks of going "light" on health support. Our allies may provide some portions of deployed military health care, but we cannot assume that this will be sufficient. Also, past experience has shown that CF members have unique medical requirements that only a CF military medical system with Canadian practitioners can meet. Moreover, from a moral point of view, we have an obligation to provide care to our own. The question then becomes, for whom will we be providing care?

FUTURE MILITARY HEALTH CLIENTS

There are indications that the Canadian population is changing; therefore, it is reasonable to assume that CF recruits of the future will have some different social and psychological characteristics from their predecessors. Leitch et al have postulated that future warfighters will "come from homes where changes in social values and lifestyles have made them physically and psychologically 'softer' than their forefathers."[29] Demographic projections for Canada indicate that the CF will be drawing its members from a somewhat smaller population base coming from several distinct "tribes" with attitudes and experiences that will shape both their health care needs and their response to health challenges such as injury and the psychological effects of operations. Imagine the effect of a permanent disability, such as a limb loss, on a soldier with a high need for autonomy and control of his (or her) destiny, what Michael Adams calls the "Autonomous Post-Materialists."[30] In addition to the expected anger and shock such an injury inflicts on any patient, this cohort of young Canadians has attitudes that will heighten that response. Canadian military health care will need to prepare itself to deal with these attitudes, the divergent attitudes of the other tribes, and the consequent psychological and psychiatric challenges their involvement in combat operations will bring.

Another change in attitudes from the past is that our society has come to expect military success at the smallest possible cost. The low mortality figures in the first Gulf War (148 for the US, 0 for Canada) have engendered both an expectation of and a low tolerance for combat deaths.[31] Failure to provide adequate health services to achieve this end would not be tolerated by the Canadian public. The response of Canadians to combat casualties in Afghanistan demonstrates a degree of acceptance by the Canadian public of "the cost of doing business" but it is uncertain what limits there are to such forbearance. It is clear from the Croatia Board of Inquiry and the continuing public concern with Gulf War related illnesses, that at certain times in the past Canadians have had little tolerance for a health system that does not respond promptly and adequately to the health concerns of CF members.

To address these issues, the CF Health Services and the US Military Health Services have learned similar lessons, albeit in slightly different ways, about what has now come to be known as Force Health Protection (FHP) and what is expected of modern military medical support. In summary those lessons are:

1) **Improved Communication.** There is a need for clear communication of risk about both combat, infectious, and environmental health hazards and treatments such as immunizations and disease prophylaxis. This need has been shown by such diverse issues as anthrax immunization and malaria prophylaxis with

mefloquine. This communication strategy must not only inform the potential patients, but the wider community as well.

2) **Health Surveillance.**   There is a clear opportunity in the information age to improve the epidemiological knowledge of both the rates of diseases and the potential cause factors.

3) **Health Records:** Linked with lesson number two is the need for improved medical record keeping and operational exposure data.   The hope (as yet unrealized by any system) is that the computerized medical record will achieve the needed comprehensiveness, timeliness and accessibility.

4) **Biomedical Research.** The need for military healthcare research above and beyond civilian healthcare research base is clear. From improved counter-measures to the Chemical Biological, Nuclear Radiological (CBNR) threat to improved combat casualty care with the products of the ongoing biotechnology revolution, research for specific military medical issues is imperative.

5) **Interagency Coordination.** The coordination of care between the Regular Force, the civilian health care system, and Veterans Affairs Canada (VAC) has never been more important. Disease and injury effects do not end with the end of deployment or even a service career. The need for a seamless transition to non-military caregivers is clear.[32]

These lessons have been incorporated into existing and planned changes to the CF Health Services,[33] but the trends in the need for client focus and information management these lessons represent will intensify with the increasing education level of CF members and the increasing availability of health information on the internet. The day of the all-knowing health practitioner doling out unquestioned wisdom is gone.

FUTURE CASUALTY TRENDS

Both the RMA and Operations Other than War (OOTW) will have major effects on casualty rates, and these effects will pose challenges to existing military medical planning procedures and doctrine. For years NATO has used Supreme Headquarters Allied Powers Europe (SHAPE) planning figures to estimate casualty rates and hence the need for military medical health support. The SHAPE figures were based on a large conventional conflict in Central Europe, but as the Balkan peacekeeping mission and the first Gulf War have shown, these planning figures are inadequate to the task of predicting health care needs in modern military operations. Overestimation of need unnecessarily increases the logistics load and may lead planners to forego certain force package options. Underestimation puts deployed forces at undue risk. The international force (IFOR) mission to the Former Yugoslavia afforded the opportunity to compare SHAPE planning figures to actual data (from the EPINATO database[34]) based on the experience of the Multinational Division Southwest (MND(SW)) deployed to the Former Yugoslavia, January to September 1998. In summary, disease occurrence was approximately 70 percent of the planning figures and the non-battle injury rate was five times the projected rate.[35]

The key issue here is that the type of casualty seen and the diseases suffered were completely different than what was initially planned for.[36] Modern peacekeeping and peacemaking operations produce a need for medical care that is different in both scope and magnitude from traditional warfighting. Unless these needs are accurately predicted and planned for, an unnecessary logistic load on the overall operation and the possibility of deploying inappropriate medical care specialty mixes may result. In an excellent review of recent military operations and the resulting casualty experience, Gouge has analyzed the casualty experience of several recent military operations.

In Afghanistan, Soviet Forces demonstrated once again the value of rapid evacuation to definitive surgical care. This created a need for more intensive care beds in-theatre. They also demonstrated the value of moving surgical teams closer to the fighting, a strategy that reduced the "died of wounds" (DOW) rate from 4.3 to 2 percent.[37] Yet, as we have seen, without appropriate preventive medicine practices, medical resources can be overwhelmed by disease casualties.[38]

In the Falklands War, the UK lacked air superiority and this impeded helicopter casualty evacuation. The planning models for this war used Second World War data and woefully underestimated the number of burn casualties that would be encountered in a sea borne assault force, particularly if ships came under attack. Yet, Forward Surgical Teams were used to great effect and again demonstrated that quick surgical care saves lives.[39]

The medical plan for the US Panama mission involved an immediate evacuation policy (zero days of holding in theatre). Casualties were treated by Forward Surgical Teams in Panama, and then promptly air evacuated to San Antonio, Texas. Despite the six-hour flight, only two of the 258 evacuees died enroute, and evacuation was not judged to be a contributory factor to their deaths.[40]

The first Gulf War campaign was clearly affected by Combat Medical Support considerations. Major ground operations were delayed until sufficient medical resources were in place and the enormous casualty estimates (as high as 40,000) resulted in two hospital ships, 63 hospitals and 18,000 beds being deployed into theatre. Despite all the preparations, medical vehicles were unable to keep up with the armoured advance, and the doctrinally imposed tiered evacuation system proved to be inefficient and essentially was ignored. The US Army Medical Department (AMEDD) was challenged by the vast distances involved, the speed of the attack, and the number of enemy prisoners of war and refugees. It was concluded that Forward Surgical Teams, Combat Stress Control teams and combat lifesavers were beneficial; however, the 60 bed MASH proved too large and too slow for its doctrinal role.[41]

The US experience in Somalia was quite different from the Canadian experience. The disastrous Army Ranger raid into Mogadishu demonstrated the enormous difficulties in handling casualties in an urban warfare setting. It also showed the need for the US Air Force to develop the Critical Care Augmentation Team (CCAT) which deals with stabilized (more critical) as opposed to the more traditional stable patient in an air evacuation.[42]

The US experience in Bosnia mirrors the Canadian experience. In such a theatre, combat injuries are too infrequent to improve or even maintain the experience level of deployed surgeons. Telemedicine proved useful only for transmitting x-rays to be read by a radiologist as none were deployed in-theatre.[43]

In summary, it appears that future conflict will produce highly variable casualty rates and morbidity patterns. This will make the planning of adequate medical support for operations extremely difficult. There is no evident casualty pattern that can be discerned from recent experience or historical records. Nevertheless, it is clear that rapid surgical treatment of wounded combatants as close as possible to the point of wounding saves lives. Air evacuation of severely wounded personnel prior to definitive treatment can be carried out with the provision of adequate onboard equipment and expertise, thus limiting the need for extensive in-theatre bed space and a large medical logistic footprint.[44]

The lessons of the continuing need for preventive medicine will undoubtedly be learned and re-learned, as the changing nature of combat will not fundamentally change the biology of infectious disease risk to deployed forces. The use of biological warfare by some combatants would change the nature of the risk but not the biology. The challenge of providing medical care to military personnel in difficult-to-predict scenarios may seem insurmountable, but new technology may provide some answers.

EFFECTS OF NEW TECHNOLOGY ON BATTLEFIELD MEDICINE

The effects of the information revolution on health care will continue, as health care personnel at all levels will have increased access to the medical literature and to patient-specific information. Health planners will be able to have a better picture of what is going on in operations and of what demands will be made of the military health care system. Furthermore, telemedicine will extend health care expertise further out onto the battlefield.

Advances in the control of bleeding, resuscitation fluids and artificial blood will change the dynamic of trauma care, enabling first responders to do more and allowing more severely wounded patients to be stabilized for transport. Miniaturized medical equipment, individualized monitors, and communication technologies will increase the efficiency and effectiveness of triage.

New, single dose multivalent vaccines,[45] genomic-based[46] therapeutics, and new antibiotics will provide more and better response to traditional battlefield infectious diseases and the CBRN threat. Improved diagnostics that will allow for rapid identification of chemical and biological threats will facilitate treatment and prophylaxis.

Genomics will provide the health care system with an increased ability to screen for disease and the propensity for disease; however, without concomitant treatment capabilities this may pose ethical and legal challenges to military medicine. For example, if we know a potential recruit is susceptible to certain diseases, which he or she will only be exposed to under certain very specific combat conditions, can we deny him or her entry to the CF? If we allow that person to enroll are we ethically obliged to prevent him or her from being exposed to such combat conditions? Since all immunization schemes pose some risk to the recipients, what are the ethics of immunizing for a disease threat that will only occur if others choose to violate accepted norms of war? How are these risks balanced against needs of the organization to maintain combat capability and the often unpredictable risk of exposure to the causative agent? Anthrax is the current best example of this problem, but smallpox and other diseases loom on the horizon.

IMPLICATIONS FOR THE CF HEALTH SERVICES

Future trends in military operations, civilian health care, the RMA and technological changes in providing health care will have profound effects on the provision of health services to the CF. The implications for the CF care system will be summarized here.

Health care provider shortages in Canada will continue and the CF will need to use the civilian health care system for both primary care and specialist support in garrison and to receive casualties sent home from operations. The mix of providers within the CF will change, as medics and nurses will assume roles traditionally exclusive to physicians.

On the battlefield, non-traditional providers such as combat medics, who can provide immediate life sustaining care to his fellow combatants, will play an increasing role. The linear evacuation of casualties will evolve to a "hub and spoke" model, i.e., intense initial stabilization will occur very close to the point of wounding. The combat medic will accomplish this with some of the new casualty treatment technologies that are "on the horizon." Alternatively, rapidly deployed medical teams with "brilliant capabilities"[47] will fly to the casualty who will then be directly evacuated to definitive surgical care. This process will bring into question the existence and role of the Field Ambulance, as it currently exists. Small forward surgical teams with only one operating table and no patient holding capacity will be necessary to effect timely care. Casualty evacuation by vertical lift (helicopters or tilt-rotor aircraft) will become increasingly important in order to provide timely and effective care on the dispersed battlefield of tomorrow. Mass casualties are unlikely and thus the deployment of the entire field hospital as it currently exists is unlikely, and modules of the field hospital similar to the current Advanced Surgical Centres (ASCs) will become the norm.

The nature and intensity of peacetime and peacekeeping operations argues for the use of the Reserves to furnish the maximum possible number of medical specialists (surgeons, anesthetists, etc.) for the CF. Current casualty rates and in-garrison patient demands are insufficient to maintain clinical competence in the Regular Force without almost continuous exposure to a pool of civilian patients. However, the current limitations of the employment of Reserves under the National Defence Act, which in effect precludes compulsory call-out, make this a risky if not impossible policy to follow for Canada.

Biotechnology advances will allow the CF Health Services to screen for many more diseases and disease potentials, and advances in information technology hold the promise of better population surveillance and ultimately better care. While this potentially will ensure a fitter and healthier force, there are problems with the application of these technologies. These advances will pose legal, moral and ethical challenges in determining member fitness to serve.

Modern technology offers some hope for diminishing the traditional infectious disease scourges of the battlefield, but history and recent Canadian experience show that we must be constantly vigilant to the threat of disease. Commanders will need to plan for optimum casualty management that emphasizes speed of treatment and rapid evacuation over the ability to handle masses of casualties in a linear tiered fashion. To ensure optimum casualty management the CF will need to develop even closer links with its primary health care partner - the US.

Finally, while it might be tempting to go extremely light on CF medical support and plan for it to be provided by our allies, this is a risky and immoral stance to take. If Canada wishes to put its military personnel in harm's way, then it must be prepared to sustain them medically with appropriate Canadian military health care support. To achieve this goal, health care providers must continue to engage those involved in operations in a dialogue on the need for and the limitations of health care in maintaining operational capability. But, if we accept that "Military Healthcare is too important to be left entirely to military healthcare professionals,"[48] then the senior leadership of DND must understand these issues if they are to ensure that CF personnel receive the kind of care Canadians demand both now and in the future.

NOTES

1   Canada, Department of National Defence (DND), *Shaping the Future of the Canadian Forces: A Strategy for 2020* (Ottawa: DND, 1999), Part II, pp. 1-12, available at http://www.vcds.dnd.ca/cds/strategy2k/s2k06_e.asp#1.

2   Desmond Morton, "Military Medicine and State Medicine: Historical Notes on the Canadian Army Medical Corps in the First World War 1914-1919," in David C. Naylor, ed. *Canadian Health Care and the State* (Montreal & Kingston: McGill-Queen's Univ. Press, 1992), 39.

3   Ronald F. Bellamy and Craig H. Llewellyn, "Preventable Casualties: Rommel's Flaw, Slim's Edge," *Army* 40, no. 5 (May 1990), 52-6.

4   Lester W. Grau and William A. Jorgensen, "Beaten by the Bugs: The Soviet-Afghan War Experience," *Military Review* 77, no. 6 (Nov-Dec 1997), 30-7.

5   Personal Communication Director General Health Services (DGHS), BGen L. Mathieu, to Col D.A. Salisbury.

6   DND, *Project Rx2000: An Update* (Canadian Forces Health Services: Ottawa, 2002).

7   DND, *Standing Committee on Operational Medicine Review, Phase One Final Report* (DGHS: Ottawa, 2001).

8   A.M. Smith, "All Bleeding Stops Eventually," *United States Naval Institute. Proceedings* 127, no. 11 (November 2001), 68-71

9   Smith, "All Bleeding Stops Eventually," 68-71.

10   G. Cecchine, et al., *Army Medical Strategy: Issues for the Future* (Santa Monica, CA: RAND Corp., 2001).

11   Commission on the Future of Health Care in Canada, *Building on Values: The Future of Health Care in Canada – Final Report* (Ottawa: np, 2002). Available at http://www.hc-sc.gc.ca/english/pdf/romanow/pdfs/HCC_Final_Report.pdf.

12   See for example R.G. Mclellan, *The Care of Injured Personnel and their Families Review* (Ottawa: DND, 1997); L.Thomas, *The Thomas Report* (Ottawa: DND, 2000); Standing Committee on National Defence and Veterans Affairs (SCONDVA), *Moving Forward: A Strategic Plan for Quality of Life Improvements in the Canadian Forces* (Ottawa,1998); and DND, *Final Report: Board of Inquiry - Croatia* (Ottawa: DND, 2000). Note that the Board's Report was on the DND website for some time after its release. It has since been removed, and virtually nothing of the Board's work is now available on the DND website

13   DND, *Project Rx2000: An Update*.

14   Commission on the Future of Health Care in Canada, *Building on Values*.

15   The Spectrum of Care for the Canadian Forces is generally based on the coverage of the Public Service Health Plan. The intent is to provide to CF members with a comparable spectrum of care to what the majority of Canadians would be provided with in their home provinces. There is no universal coverage plan in Canada.

16   R.A. Leitch, H.R. Champion, and J.F. Navein, "The Future of U.S. Military Health Services in a Time of Great Change," in *Landpower Essay Series* (Arlington, VA : Institute of Land Warfare,1998), 1-8.

17   A.M. Smith, "Military Medicine: Not the Same as Practising Medicine in the Military," *Armed Forces and Society* 18, no. 4 (Summer 1992), 585.

18   Canadian Institute of Health Information (CIHI), *Health Care in Canada 2002* (Ottawa: CIHI, Statistics Canada, 2002), 123.

19   S. Beaty, "The Revolution in Military Medical Affairs," *Parameters* 27, no. 4 (Winter 1997-8), 60-72.

20   J.J Dougherty, "Operational Medical Support for the Tip of the Spear: The Heart of Air Force Special Operations Forces (AFSOF) Medicine," *Aerospace Power Journal* 15, no. 4 (Winter 2001), 27-33.

21   Canadian Forces Search and Rescue (SAR) Techs are trained in multiple skills including parachuting, survival, mountain climbing and SCUBA diving. For the last several years they have been trained in paramedic procedures at the Justice Institute in British Columbia where they receive similar training to advanced paramedics in the Ambulance Service of BC.

22   See for example Smith, "Military Medicine," 576-91; Leitch, "The Future of U.S. Military Health Services in a Time of Great Change," 1-8; and Cecchine et al., *Army Medical Strategy*.

23   DND, *Advancing with Purpose: The Army Strategy* (Ottawa: DND, 2002), 1-32.

24   Dougherty, "Operational Medical Support for the Tip of the Spear," 27-33.

25   See for example Leitch, "The Future of U.S. Military Health Services in a Time of Great Change"; and J.R. Blaker, *Understanding the Revolution in Military Affairs: A Guide to America's 21ᵈ Century Defense* (Washington, DC: Progressive Policy Institute,1997).

26   Smith, "All Bleeding Stops Eventually," 68-71.

27   See Allan D. English, *The Cream of the Crop: Canadian Aircrew 1939-1945* (Montreal & Kingston:McGill-Queen's University Press, 1996), 61-130 for a more detailed discussion of these issues.

28   Cecchine et al., *Army Medical Strategy*.

29   Leitch, "The Future of U.S. Military Health Services in a Time of Great Change," 1-8.

30   Michael Adams, *Sex in the Snow: Canadian Social Values at the End of the Millennium* (Toronto: Penguin Books 1998), 42-57.

31   M.W. Alvis, "Understanding the Role of Casualties in U.S. Peace Operations," in *Landpower Essay Series* (Arlington, VA : Institute of Land Warfare,1998), 1-16.

32   J.F. Mazzuchi, et al., "Force Health Protection:10 Years of Lessons Learned by the Department of Defense," *Military Medicine* 167, no. 3 (March 2002), 179-85.

33   DND, *Project Rx2000: An Update;* and DND, *Standing Committee on Operational Medicine Review, Phase One Final Report*.

34   EPINATO is a medical database system now widely in use in the alliance to collect near real time disease and injury data on deployed forces in a particular geographic area.

35   P.I. Rafaelli, "Medical Implications of Recent Strategic Political and Military Changes," *Journal of the Royal Naval Medical Service* 85, no. 1 (Spring 1999) 25-30.

36   Personal Observation. Colonel Salisbury was Deputy Force Surgeon for IFOR from June to December 1996.

37   S.F. Gouge, *Combat Health Support of the Transformation Force in 2015* (Carlisle Barracks, PA: US Army War College, 2001). Statistics from p. 11.

38   Grau and Jorgensen, "Beaten by the Bugs," 30-7.

39   Gouge, *Combat Health Support of the Transformation Force in 2015*, 11.

40   Ibid., 12.

41   Ibid., 13.

42   Gouge, *Combat Health Support of the Transformation Force in 2015*, 14; and P.K. Carlton, "New Millennium, New Mind-Set: The Air Force Medical Services in the Air Expeditionary Era," *Aerospace Power Journal* 15, no. 4 (Winter 2001), 8-13.

43   Gouge, *Combat Health Support of the Transformation Force in 2015*, 15.

44   Carlton, "New Millennium, New Mind-Set," 8-13.

45   Multivalent vaccines are vaccines that can be used against multiple infectious agents. For example, the current first vaccine in Canada for children is a pentavalent vaccine against Diphtheria, Pertussis, Tetanus, Polio and H. influenza.

46   Genomics or the study of human genetics will eventually enable therapies to be specifically tailored to the genetic makeup of the individual patient. Current therapies are based on what medical science judges is best for the majority or the average patient.

47   Beaty, "The Revolution in Military Medical Affairs," 60-72.

48   Leitch, "The Future of U.S. Military Health Services in a Time of Great Change," 1-8.

CHAPTER 2

THREATS TO OPERATIONAL FORCE HEALTH PROTECTION

Colonel Jean-Robert Bernier

...the tricks of marching and of shooting and the game called strategy constitute only a part – the minor, although picturesquely appealing part – of the tragedy of war. They are only the terminal operations engaged in by those remnants of the armies which have survived the camp epidemics. These have often determined victory or defeat before the generals know where they are going to place the headquarters mess.

H. Zinsser[1]

INTRODUCTION

An important lesson from history is that in most military operations the majority of casualties (and often deaths) have resulted from disease and non-battle injuries (DNBI) rather than from hostile action. Therefore, the scale of DNBI casualties has often decided or had a major impact on to the outcome of conflicts.[2] Such casualties have continued to affect Canadian Forces (CF) operations and those of our major allies in recent years, yet most are unnecessary and preventable. Over the past decade, a number of developments, such as deployment-related health problems and the threat of nuclear, biological and chemical (NBC) weapons, have helped to re-focus attention on the lesson from history about DNBI, and major enhancements have been made to CF operational health protection capabilities and awareness as a result. These enhancements have included better capabilities to protect CF members against infectious diseases, other environmental and industrial hazards, deployment-related stress, and NBC agents.[3] The primary role and importance of commanders in the application of health protection measures is also well recognized by the senior CF leadership, but several problems persist or are developing that threaten the CF's ability to protect its members from deployment-related hazards. If not adequately mitigated or resolved, some of these problems could degrade or neutralize some health protection capabilities and potentially result in grave consequences to individual health and to operational success. This chapter argues that, despite recent capability advances, the ability to protect the health of members of the CF is threatened by societal developments and adverse command factors.

It is generally accepted that armed forces should strive for casualty prevention rather than treatment after onset of illness or injury,[4] and it is to preventive measures that the term "health protection" will refer here. Paradoxically, however, command and staff attention to medical issues has historically tended to focus primarily on casualty treatment and evacuation rather than on prevention.[5] Yet, casualties result not only in personnel loss, but also in the expenditure of limited medical and evacuation resources and a need to train, transport and integrate replacement personnel. Given the relatively small scale of many CF operations, the loss of key individuals or of single aircraft for medical evacuation (from a ship for example) may have a significant operational impact. This chapter will examine force health protection by first asserting the operational importance of force health protection and the ongoing consequences of inadequate command attention to its application. A summary of current CF health protection efforts and capabilities is then described, and will be followed by a discussion of societal and command factors that hinder their effectiveness. Finally, a conclusion will summarize concerns and propose general measures to mitigate them.

IMPORTANCE OF FORCE HEALTH PROTECTION

> …soldiers have rarely won wars. They more often mop up after the barrage of epidemics.
>
> H. Zinsser[6]

Force health protection is critically important for operational, strategic, and ethical reasons. Operationally, the CF health protection has recently focused on low-level chemical and radiological exposures, but these hazards are usually of relatively low health significance.[7] Most operational casualties have been and continue to be caused by infectious diseases, temperature extremes, and physical injuries.[8] There is an extensive record of the disastrous effects of these factors on military operations and "the difficulty is not to find evidence, but to select from the dreadful abundance."[9] While many are aware that 80 percent of Napoleon's losses during his Russian campaign were caused by infectious diseases and exposure,[10] fewer know that Field Marshal Rommel's neglect of basic field hygiene and sanitation was a major contributor to his ultimate defeat in North Africa. The preventable diseases that plagued his Afrika Korps troops cost him, temporarily or permanently, a force equal to twice his average strength. General Slim commanding the British 14th Army in Burma, on the other hand, reversed the steady destruction of his army from disease by rigorously enforcing health protection measures and he ultimately inflicted on the Japanese Army its greatest defeat.[11]

One might expect that the availability of modern field hygiene and prophylactic medications over the past few decades would effectively mitigate such operational hazards, but, in the absence of adequate command attention to force health protection, this has not always been the case. For example, in Vietnam, US forces suffered annual averages of about 400 DNBI casualties per 1,000 soldiers compared to 100 battle casualties per 1,000 soldiers. Egyptian forces suffered 20,000 heat-related deaths during the 1967 Six-Day War, and inadequate British planning during the Falklands War contributed to 109 cold injuries out of 777 total casualties.[12] During the Soviet occupation of Afghanistan in the 1980s, poor field hygiene and sanitation resulted in 67 percent of the deployed force of 620,000 being hospitalized at some point for disease.[13] Of the 28,000 US troops hospitalized during the first Gulf War, less than 1000 were for combat-related injuries, and only 1000 of the 8000 medical evacuations were combat-related.[14] And largely because of poor compliance with protective measures, British forces suffered very high malaria casualty rates during operations in Sierra Leone in 2000,[15] and several major infectious disease outbreaks have afflicted the crews of allied warships in the past few years.[16] Similarly, a severe viral respiratory disease rendered the British field hospital in Bagram non-functional during operations in Afghanistan in 2002[17] and 44 percent of US Marines who went ashore in Liberia in 2003 suffered a potentially life-threatening form of malaria.[18] This small sample, which does not include the long-term toll of suffering and personnel loss resulting from operational stress injuries, demonstrates the ongoing impact of DNBI and the need for careful attention to force health protection.

A few examples illustrate that the CF also continues to experience or risk suffering preventable operational casualties through inadequate command understanding of or attention to health protection issues. During the 2000 East Timor mission, 46 percent of the CF contingent in Dili was infected with potentially life-threatening Dengue fever. This extremely high rate of mosquito-borne infection occurred because the commander did not apply a medically recommended preventive countermeasure and compliance with other recommended measures was inadequately enforced. Co-located foreign contingents had better compliance records and did not suffer a single case of Dengue fever.[19] During Operation Apollo (Afghanistan and the Persian Gulf (Arabian Gulf) region) in 2002, planning and execution shortfalls led to the loss or non-application of important medical NBC defensive measures.[20] In addition, during the theatre activation phase of Operation Athena in the summer of 2003, a deployed junior commander in Kabul, Afghanistan was aware that malaria prophylaxis was medically recommended, but advised other deploying personnel that it was not necessary.[21] Furthermore, despite extensive support from the senior CF leadership for the establishment of a deployable industrial hygiene capability, its deployment for the conduct of air quality and other health hazard assessments was initially opposed by elements of the Joint Staff.[22] The same summer, a gastro-intestinal disease epidemic struck a large proportion of the CF contingent deployed to Zgon, Bosnia.[23]

Besides an operational impact, strategic consequences may also result from inadequate health protection measures. For example, if CF measures are inferior to those of major allies (for example against drug- or vaccine-preventable diseases), CF elements may be perceived as a weak link in a coalition to the extent that their vulnerability would be increased and operational reliability reduced. Inadequate health protection against contagious diseases (naturally spread or spread by biological weapons) could also result in the unprotected force presenting a positive threat to allied forces, the host nation's population, and the homeland. In recent years, infected military personnel have imported various infectious diseases that could have or did present a threat to civilian populations.[24] If an imported infectious agent is contagious or is acquired by a suitable domestic insect or animal vector, it could result in the introduction and spread of a new disease to North America with general adverse health and economic consequences.   In such circumstances, host nationals, allies, and Canadian health authorities might perceive CF elements as a public health threat.

Finally, it is morally, legally, and politically unacceptable to Canadians and to political and military leaders for CF members to be deployed with inadequate health protection measures.[25] This was reflected in the public debate concerning the availability of anthrax vaccine to CF elements deploying to the Persian Gulf during Operation Determination in 1998, the findings and recommendations of the Croatia Board of Inquiry, and recent national interest in the adequacy of smallpox vaccine stocks and the military vaccination policy. Unlike civilian workers, CF members cannot refuse lawful orders to perform dangerous or deadly operational activities. Commanders, therefore, arguably have a greater moral duty than other employers to ensure that all possible measures are taken to mitigate health risks. As Slim noted, "The most important thing about a commander is his effect on morale."[26] It is essential for morale, recruiting, retention, and general institutional credibility that CF members and the public perceive military commanders to be doing all that is possible to protect their subordinates from preventable illness and injury. It is also CF policy that commanders comply with the health and safety requirements of the Canada Labour Code except where precluded by operational exigencies.[27] And financially, the CF and government retain indefinite responsibility for the care and compensation of injured or ill members.[28]

BACKGROUND AND CURRENT CF CAPABILITIES

The CF has the potential to avoid most preventable DNBI since its technical health protection expertise and capabilities are now among the best of any armed forces in the world.[29] This is, however, a recent development. During the Cold War, the focus on Western Europe and the infrequency of expeditionary missions to underdeveloped regions of the world presented few major industrial or environmental health hazards to the CF. There was thus a relatively limited CF preventive medicine capability requirement and much of the small health protection staff's efforts were directed at in-garrison and NBC health protection.[30] With the post-Cold War force reductions of the early 1990s, the small health protection staff was further reduced. Unfortunately for the CF, this reduction coincided with a marked increase in expeditionary deployments to regions with significant industrial and natural environmental hazards such as tropical infectious diseases, poor transportation and industrial infrastructure, and inadequate industrial contamination standards.[31] At the same time, this period was characterized by great interest in possible links between deployment-related exposures and ill health reported by veterans of the first Gulf War and other operations.

As invariably happens when preventive health efforts are neglected, a series of health concerns arose. These concerns contributed to the establishment of several independent reviews including the Chief of Review Services Report on the CF Medical Service, the McLellan Report, the Thomas Report, and the Report of the Croatia Board of Inquiry. Each identified significant health protection deficiencies and almost all of their recommendations are being funded and implemented through the Rx2000 Project, an expanded Force Health Protection organization, and the Environmental and Industrial Health Hazard Project.[32] These enhancements are providing the CF with a very high standard of expertise in health hazard assessment and mitigation, military operational medicine, health intelligence, health surveillance and epidemiology, health promotion, occupational and environmental health, communicable disease control, industrial hygiene, preventive medicine, and mental health screening and management. Medical staff, however, has no authority to enforce the application of many capabilities or health protection measures since most require command direction, non-medical administrative controls, or engineering mitigation measures. These are command prerogatives and responsibilities, and to address these prerogatives and responsibilities Deputy Chief of the Defence Staff (DCDS) Directions for International Operations (DDIO) provided detailed policy direction concerning protection against health hazards.[33] Furthermore, a multi-disciplinary Environmental Health and Safety Committee (EHSC), chaired, appropriately, by J3 International on the DCDS staff, was also established to determine and coordinate necessary health protection measures for deployed CF elements.

OBSTACLES TO EFFECTIVE FORCE HEALTH PROTECTION

Despite these encouraging capability developments, several societal and command factors hinder their full application. Health protection is being progressively hindered or complicated by a cultural tendency in favour of the primacy of individual interests and privacy, health risk misperception, and suspicion and distrust of science and authority. It is also degraded by shortcomings in leader training and awareness, command authority, doctrine, and planning. These issues will be addressed next.

Societal Factors

Individual rights. Since the promulgation of the Charter of Rights and Freedoms, Canadian society is commonly perceived to emphasize, more than ever, informed consent for medical interventions and the supremacy of individual autonomy and rights over those of institutions or the collective interest. Even during a deadly contagious disease outbreak, such as the 2003 Severe Acute Respiratory Syndrome (SARS) epidemic in Toronto, there was considerable public controversy over the violation of individual liberties (such as the imposition of quarantine) necessary to protect the public health. Similarly, during the 2001-02 influenza season, the Ontario government declined to enforce mandatory influenza vaccination of defiant paramedics as authorized by the Ambulance Act even though infected unvaccinated personnel could pose a deadly hazard to vulnerable immune-suppressed patients.[34]

The culture from which CF members are now recruited is widely perceived to be relatively self-centred.[35] Military service is considered by many to be an occupation rather than a vocation, and current CF training and orientation may not adequately instill military values such as self-sacrifice and the primacy of mission accomplishment.[36] The potential threat posed to the military mission or to others by individual failure to accept or apply health protection measures (such as drugs or vaccines) may no longer be considered sufficient justification for making them mandatory. Therefore, there may be a progressive reluctance to accept medical countermeasures against NBC or tropical disease since the threat and mission impact of exposure to such agents depend on unpredictable factors that cannot always be accurately quantified or predicted. Finally, the modification of the universality of service principle and the consequent retention of non- or partly-deployable personnel, while reasonable and compassionate, may result in a reduced personnel pool for sustainment. The potentially increased operational tempo for those who remain fully deployable may have adverse effects on their morale, family stress, and mental health. Another societal factor that affects force health protection is privacy.

Privacy. To assess an individual's health risk or to determine if illness is related to preceding exposure, medical epidemiological staff routinely require access to individual health records, accurate exposure data, and accurate individual location- and time-specific deployment history. These data are also necessary to permit the identification of unusual illness patterns among groups and their relationship to exposures or deployments. The identification of such patterns permits the implementation of appropriate exposure and illness prevention and control measures. The results of epidemiological health surveillance are also necessary to assess the CF's general health status and to guide CF efforts and policies concerning health promotion, health protection, treatment, training, medical standards, and recruit screening. Trend identification may be extremely urgent if a dangerous exposure results in a time-sensitive treatment window, such as a biological attack with a treatable but rapidly fatal disease agent.

Epidemiological research must comply with certain guidelines that include review of the protocol by an ethics board and, in some cases, study-specific informed consent of each person whose data is to be examined. Although this requirement does not currently apply to routine health surveillance, newly proposed Canadian health research guidelines may make such routine surveillance subject to the same requirements.[37] Should these requirements be imposed on routine health surveillance, they will significantly delay and increase the difficulty with which deployment-related illness trends, patterns, and exposure-illness linkages could be assessed. Such requirements could reduce the CF's ability to identify, mitigate or eliminate harmful practices or exposures in a timely manner and to optimally tailor subsequent health protection and promotion efforts. Increasingly restrictive privacy regulations also hinder or delay epidemiological staff access to medical records and individual contact information.[38] These regulations hinder health surveillance efforts and the assessment of exposure-illness relationships. They could also delay necessary medical interventions for those who previously experienced a deployment-related exposure that is subsequently linked to a health concern. Finally, the multitude of health-related questionnaires and surveys administered over the past few years has naturally led some commanders to wish to restrict the burden placed on their troops. While this provides some short-term relief to individual CF members, an inability to acquire health-related data will hinder the identification and assessment of physical and mental health trends and needs, as well as the appropriate modification of health protection and promotion efforts and policies.

Health risk misperception. Despite extensive evidence to the contrary and the consistent conclusions of all expert bodies that have examined the issues, many persons still believe that there is a unique Gulf War Syndrome caused by an unknown environmental exposure and that medical countermeasures such as anthrax vaccine or pyridostigmine bromide are unsafe.[39] The spread of rumours among troops that some medical remedies are not safe is not a new problem as Slim observed about malaria prophylaxis in his command, "…there was the usual whispering campaign among troops that greets every new remedy – the drug would render them impotent – so, often the little tablet was not swallowed.[40] And yet the problem of rumours degrading the effectiveness of force health protection has been increased because the internet and mass media provide individuals with a multitude of instantaneous information sources (factual or otherwise) concerning health hazards. North Americans also generally tend to overestimate negligible health risks while underestimating severe ones, and there is a natural tendency for them to attribute unexplained symptoms to an unusual preceding exposure. The resulting misperceptions are often initiated or reinforced by uncritical, exaggerated and sensational media reporting that bears little relationship to the actual magnitude of the health hazard, does not distinguish between allegation and scientific evidence, or deliberately misleads. Misperceptions can also be reinforced by judicial rulings on cause-and-effect relationships that, while legally reasonable if the court standard only requires the establishment of a subjective likelihood, are incongruent with scientific standards to demonstrate causation. Other authorities may assume causation unless proved otherwise. The US Congress has, for example, authorized ill veterans exposed to herbicides such as Agent Orange to be compensated without any causal link having been established between exposure and illness. While the objective scientific reality remains unchanged, many persons will accept contrary judicial, political, or media declarations.[41]

Distrust. Aggravating such misperceptions are the broader societal phenomena of distrust of objective science in favour of subjective assessments and feelings, an unrealistic desire for and expectation of zero risk, and a distrust of institutional authorities.[42] Jon Franklin, a Pulitzer Prize-winning science writer in the United States, has written, "What we are seeing, in the press and in our society, is nothing less than the deconstruction of the Enlightenment and its principle institution, which is science."[43] Both the Croatia and Somalia inquiries noted the development of distrust of the CF leadership during the 1990s, particularly with respect to stress-related illness.[44] Some of this distrust extended to CF medical authorities, who face the dilemma of being bound to do what is best for individual patients while at the same time having a duty to conform to potentially conflicting CF operational requirements.[45] Distrust among some has also been aggravated by the fact that several CF medical countermeasures against NBC or tropical disease threats, while authorized for use by Health Canada, are not licensed in Canada. This situation will necessarily continue because the Canadian market for such rarely used products is too small to make the considerable expense of obtaining a license worth the cost to pharmaceutical companies. Although they have well-established safety and efficacy data and are usually licensed in other western countries, a misperception exists among some that these products are "experimental." There is also little recognition that perfect safety is unattainable for any medical product and that all medical interventions are based on a risk versus benefit assessment. These factors may feed a misperception that medical authorities recommend and command authorities mandate the use of countermeasures based primarily on their short-term contribution to mission accomplishment, and that their long-term health effects are but secondary considerations.

Potential adverse effects of the trends listed above on health protection may include soldier non-compliance with force protection countermeasures and judicial or political decisions that restrict the CF leadership's authority to mandate them. There has already been a Senate sub-committee proposal to review the Chief of the Defence Staff's (CDS) authority to mandate medical countermeasures and a judicial decision in favour of a CF member's refusal to comply with them. When a counter-measure with a misperceived health risk is mandated, morale may suffer through a paradoxical loss of confidence in the CF leadership's concern for individual health and disciplinary situations may arise. This was demonstrated by the refusal of Sergeant Michael Kipling to submit to anthrax vaccination during Operation Determination, in the Persian Gulf (Arabian Gulf) area in 1998. Contrary to expert opinion and the assurances of US and Canadian national civilian and military health authorities, there were at the time sensational media reports of vaccine quality control concerns and possible links to symptoms reported by some veterans of the first Gulf War. Despite the unanimous position of the vaccine expert scientific and medical communities, the judge at his widely-publicized court martial hearing ruled that the vaccine lot was unsafe, that ordering Sergeant Kipling to receive it violated his Charter right to security of the person, and that the charge should not proceed.[46] The ruling was later overturned on appeal, but this appeal ruling received relatively little publicity. For some CF members, the initial ruling likely raised or confirmed suspicions that their health might be a secondary concern to senior CF command and health authorities, that government and scientific authorities in general could not be trusted, and that a critical force protection countermeasure should (and could) be avoided. The original ruling also created a precedent whereby a CF member received judicial support for disobedience of a lawful command on the basis of his personal assessment of the hazard posed by an operational force protection measure. Since military operations necessarily require acceptance of orders to perform activities that are far more hazardous than vaccination, and since there is no medical countermeasure for which there is not an opposition argument, a general application of the prece-dent would render any force operationally ineffective.

Misperception of health risk may also result in stress- or worry-related ill-ness. It is well established that, regardless of actual exposure, the suspi-cion or belief that one has experienced a harmful exposure can lead to the development or aggravation of (sometimes incapacitating) symptoms and illness.[47] There is also an extensive body of literature demonstrating that some persons who are treated like ill patients adopt such a role. The com-bat stress literature in particular indicates that soldiers treated in this manner and evacuated to rear medical facilities are highly unlikely to recover and return to duty.[48] Thus, there is a risk of contributing to the development of illness by overemphasizing, or "medicalizing," exposures of no health significance or of distressing, but non-pathological, reactions to stress. The media in particular, though generally well-meaning in seeking to enhance the safety of CF members, may paradoxically contribute to illness and injury through exaggeration or dissemination of inaccurate health risk information that leads to unnecessary worry or to non-compliance with health protection measures. The stress-illness connection was further complicated in the 1990s by a reluctance of government and insurance compensation adjudicators to accept stress-related illness or mental health problems as eligible deployment-related outcomes.[49] Since objectively-demonstrable and codified physical causes were favoured, there would have been a strong practical and psychological incentive for ill CF members to establish that symptoms were related to an identifiable and concrete exposure (such as a drug, vaccine, air or ground contaminant). These concerns emphasize the need for a sound health risk assessment, pro-active communication of accurate information (particularly of negative findings), and a strong health surveillance capability to record exposures and detect adverse individual or group health outcomes.

Another adverse effect on health protection could result from commanders focusing primarily on avoidance of low-level chemical or radiological exposures, the main concerns of the first Gulf War and Operation Harmony (Balkan Region February 1992 - December 1995) veterans and the subject of an ongoing national public debate, to the detriment of efforts to prevent the more significant threats posed by food-, water- or insect-borne infectious diseases. Similarly, although exposure to depleted uranium, for example, is of little or no health significance, there has been external pressure for the CF to devote limited pre-deployment training time to this misperceived but politically-popular issue. Risk assessment and mitigation of certain low-level chemical and radiological exposures are important to health and psychological well-being, and such hazards could potentially cause long-term health effects or heavy casualties in the event of large-scale accidental or deliberate exposure. Inadequate focus on the far greater hazards posed by infectious agents, injuries, and temperature extremes is, however, orders of magnitude more likely to result in casualties. Similarly, bivouac siting that avoids low-level chemical or radiological exposures of negligible health significance but that is tactically vulnerable may expose the force to a greater overall health threat from hostile action than from harmful contaminants.

Without strong leadership, health risk assessment, risk mitigation, and risk communication efforts, there may be a loss of confidence and compliance among CF members, resulting in increased potential for the development of psychosomatic illnesses, political concern and intervention, and greater reluctance among CF legal and command authorities to support a mandatory policy for the use of medical countermeasures. The consequent toll in unnecessary and preventable casualties could, in some circumstances, threaten not only the safety of deployed personnel but also mission success. If a voluntary consent policy was to be internally adopted or externally imposed, some operational and medical-ethical questions would arise. Would the option of refusing medical countermeasures extend to the use of chemical-containing products such as insect repellents, sunscreen, or even camouflage paint? Should medical staff deem as medically non-deployable those who refuse medical countermeasures necessary for protection against health threats in the theatre of operations? Should such persons be assigned geographic medical employment limitations and be administratively released because of limited deployability? Should and could acceptance of mandated medical countermeasures be made an explicit condition of enrolment and continued service? Is it ethical to make medical countermeasures voluntary if the threat assessment indicates that failing to have their protection may result in serious adverse consequences to individual health and to the mission? Would someone be held responsible if harm to others results or the mission fails due to the unnecessary loss of an unprotected individual incapacitated by a preventable illness?

Command Factors

> More than half the battle against disease is fought, not by doctors, but by the regimental officers...as all of us, commanders, doctors, regimental officers, staff officers, and NCOs united in the drive against sickness, results began to appear.
>
> Field Marshal Viscount Slim [50]

Command influence. Enforcement of the use of health protection measures is a command responsibility. Since Slim's campaign in Burma, many others have illustrated the critical impact of command example and support (or lack thereof) on compliance with medical force protection measures. A recent example is the British experience with voluntary anthrax vaccination during the 1998 Persian Gulf deployment. Units whose leaders clearly communicated the threat and strongly supported vaccination achieved 100 percent compliance. Those whose leaders did not had extremely poor compliance and would likely have suffered catastrophic casualties if an aerosolized anthrax attack had occurred.[51] Because of poor compliance with anti-malarial measures, British forces suffered high malaria rates during their 2000 Sierra Leone operation,[52] as did an Australian battalion in East Timor in 2000[53] and US forces after their 1993 Somalia[54] and 2003 Liberia[55] missions. Conversely, commanders can have an extremely positive impact on health as did Slim and a US Air Force Chief of Staff in the mid-1980s. After the latter simply indicated that he thought smokers should not be generals, the resulting reduction in smoking among senior US Air Force officers exceeded that of previous health promotion campaigns.[56] Finally, it has been well-established that strong leadership, unit cohesion, and realistic training are the most important factors in prevention and recovery of combat stress casualties.[57] These examples illustrate that, while competent medical capabilities and risk communication are critical to force health protection, they are supportive elements to the primary role of commanders and may be ineffective without active command support. However, consistently effective application of health protection measures is often hindered by shortcomings in middle and junior leader cadres, training, doctrine, and mission planning, as well as by the societal trends noted previously.

Leader training. The idea that senior leaders should train junior leaders in force health protection issues is at least 200 years old, as this quote from a military manual published in 1779 demonstrates: "The preservation of the soldiers health should be his [Commandant of a Regiment] first and greatest care...he must have a watchful eye over the officers of companies, that they pay the necessary attention to their men in those respects."[58] And yet in the CF, except for safety programs and theatre-specific pre-deployment health briefings, no general educational requirements have been established to ensure that deployed force health protection issues are understood at all command and staff levels. Even though DNBI usually cause more casualties than any other operational threat and their prevention depends primarily on command influence, they are not included in initial training or later professional development programs. Extensive educational efforts are, however, devoted to some other topics that have no direct relevance to force protection or military operations in general.

The Croatia Board of Inquiry, and other reports noted earlier, greatly enhanced senior level awareness of these issues and led to much-improved health protection capabilities. The reports, DDIOs, and EHSC efforts do not, however, provide CF leaders with an adequate understanding of many operationally-important health issues or with information on how to effectively ensure their subordinates understand their roles in force health protection. Senior, junior, and non-commissioned officers play the most important and direct role in influencing and enforcing compliance with health protection measures, but the examples noted earlier in this chapter clearly suggest that increased awareness has not extended to some at the operational and tactical levels. Unless education on health protection issues and requirements becomes part of professional development, commanders may be unable to appropriately weigh occupational and environmental health hazards in their overall risk assessment, to "operationalize" health protection advice, and to ensure that appropriate health protection measures are consistently applied.

Command capability imbalance. A key impediment to providing the CF with improved force health protection is the current command capability imbalance. The Pigeau-McCann command framework illustrates how command capability is dependant upon the right balance of competency, authority, and responsibility.[59] With regard to responsibility for health protection, DDIOs state: "The chain of command continues to bear the entire responsibilities of soldiers' health under their command."[60] However, this ultimate degree of responsibility is not accompanied by an equal degree of competency and authority. Competency is limited by the absence of any general service officer training in basic health protection issues. Medical advisers do not fully compensate for this shortfall since they are not usually available to all subordinate commanders, and even where available at lower levels of command, junior medical officers will generally have limited competence in military preventive medicine.

Authority is also limited given the extent of responsibility assigned. As noted above, commanders may exert an enormous positive or negative influence on health protection and many necessary measures are within their power to mandate or influence (such as general field hygiene and sanitation, hand washing, use of seat belts, enforcement of work-rest cycle and fluid intake, wearing long sleeves, use of mosquito protection, etc.). Only the CDS, however, may mandate the use of vaccines or drugs, and the societal factors noted above may progressively encourage an institutional reluctance to do so. Physical and mental stress resistance and health protection also depend on a commander's ability to influence a much broader variety of pre-, intra- and post-deployment factors such as screening and selection, adequate and realistic training, physical and mental fitness, the application of discipline, the development of trust between leader and led, quality of life and morale, and other factors related to the promotion and maintenance of health. In addition to the detrimental affects of the societal trends noted earlier, the commander's ability to influence some of these may be further hindered by over-centralization of authority in the conduct of operations and in personnel management as noted by some CF leaders. Distant centralized authorities and staffs can dictate policies and make individual personnel management decisions in areas that are relevant to the commander's ability to influence his command's health protection readiness. Commanders may, as a result, be seen as powerless by their subordinates, and the institution of oversight structures such as the Ombudsman's office may be perceived as questioning their integrity.[61] This situation may aggravate the distrust noted earlier, reduce the ability of commanders to influence or enforce compliance with health protection measures, and encourage direct appeals to central authorities if an objection to such measures arises.

Doctrine. The key force protection role of preventive medicine is emphasized by the repeated lessons of history, the obvious advantages of prevention over treatment, the importance of medical countermeasures in defence against natural and NBC hazards, and the role of medical diagnostics and health surveillance in NBC attack detection and agent identification. Slim put it this way: "…where the surgeon saved the individual life, the physician, less dramatically, saved hundreds by his preventive measures."[62] Particularly for NBC individual protection, detection, identification, and certain medical countermeasures may provide greater defensive advantages than other non-medical measures. Effective vaccines, for example, can largely obviate the need to detect, identify, don individual and collective protection, and decontaminate in a biological threat environment.[63] The role of preventive medicine is, however, reflected inconsistently or not at all in some key CF doctrine publications. The *Canadian Joint Task List*, for example, does not include force health protection, preventive medicine, or any health protection reference under the protection task, but rather lists medical issues exclusively as sustainment functions. Preventive medical countermeasures are not listed in *Canadian Forces Operations* in the chapters on Force Protection or NBC Defence. Even the chapter on Health Service Support only lists evacuation, treatment and recovery in describing its contribution to personnel effectiveness. Perhaps most importantly, *Canadian Forces Operations* only makes a passing reference to preventive medicine without acknowledging the historically critical role of casualty prevention in operational success or failure.[64]

Contractor support. Doctrinal acceptance of contractor support for certain sustainment functions does not necessarily threaten force health protection. There is, however, potential for inconsistencies and inadequacies in contractor medical screening, hygiene training and application, food handling, water quality surveillance and maintenance, and food quality. Inadequacies in any of these areas could potentially incapacitate the force through infectious disease transmission. Food handlers in particular may not have the same extensive background in hygiene training and emphasis as CF cooks, and the health of the force is particularly vulnerable to contracted food handlers' inadvertent or deliberate actions. There must thus be adequate medical input to the screening and qualifications of contracted personnel, the details and standards of contracted tasks, and the monitoring and auditing of contractor activities. Finally, stable operations may suddenly become unstable. This could result in the rapid repatriation of contracted personnel providing key health protection functions such as water quality maintenance, infectious agent vector control, or waste disposal.[65] In such cases, the force's vulnerability to disease could increase pending the deployment of qualified uniformed personnel to assume these functions.

Another force health protection issue arises from an increased reliance on contracted civilian physicians for the provision of in-garrison health care in order to enhance continuity of care and to help relieve the effects of the medical officer shortage in the CF. In the absence of a military background, some of these contracted physicians may have little understanding of the military importance of monitoring general unit health status and trends. They may also have little inclination to monitor such trends or to discuss individual or unit health status (as opposed to individual diagnoses) with commanders. Commanders have the ultimate responsibility for the health of their command and its operational effectiveness. They also have a unique ability to influence the employment of individuals and the application of and compliance with general health protection measures. It is therefore essential that, without violating medical confidentiality, commanders are kept aware of their unit's health readiness, adverse health trends and appropriate remedial actions, and measures to assist ill members' return to duty.

Operational planning. Force health protection can also be compromised if it is not an integral part of the operational planning process. For example, late inclusion of medical staff in operational planning, inadequate consideration or understanding of preventive health issues, inadequate medical representation on reconnaissance, or late deployment of key medical elements can result in inadequate health protection. These lapses can lead to DNBI from inadequate preventive preparations, the unavailability of key medical countermeasures, unresolved health concerns among deployed troops, and unforeseen deployment delays to ensure that adequate health protection measures are in place. Yet experiences from the first Gulf War in 1991 to Operation Athena in 2003 indicate that some lessons have been recorded but not learned.

For example, the Chief of Review Services' report on CF participation in the first Gulf War made observations about the inadequate consideration of medical issues in mission planning and reconnaissance.[66] Despite improvements, with the frequent inclusion of clinical and preventive medicine staff on mission reconnaissance and the routine conduct of health hazard assessments during theatre activation, published lessons from Operation Apollo also noted inadequacies in force health protection related to NBC medical countermeasures. The CF holds most of, if not the only, national supply of several very expensive and difficult-to-obtain NBC medical countermeasures. The late deployment of medical elements to Operation Apollo, however, resulted in the spoilage of a significant portion of the national supply of one of them. The force protection gaps that could result from inadequate supply of such products could lead to adverse operational, military strategic, and national consequences.

In addition to the spoilage problems, DDIO-mandated medical counter-measure briefings were not always provided to those deploying on this mission.[67] As a result, had there been a need to use certain NBC medical countermeasures during the operation, it is likely that some would have been used incorrectly resulting either in inadequate protection or adverse effects. The CF would also not have been in full compliance with its obligations for the use of unlicensed products and might have lost Health Canada's authority to import key force protection capabilities in the future. In another instance of inadequate compliance with regulations concerning the use of an unlicensed product (Mefloquine) during the Somalia mission, for example, there were significant negative repercussions on the CF.[68]

A final example of inadequate force health protection measures occurred during the 2003 Joint Support Group deployment to a Turkish industrial area in support of Operation Athena, when, despite the possibility of industrial earthquake damage and preventive medicine concerns, the deployment initially proceeded without any form of occupational health hazard assessment.[69]

CONCLUSION

Throughout military history, DNBI have resulted in adverse (and often decisive) strategic, operational, and individual health consequences. DNBI continue to cause most CF operational casualties during deployed operations and the adequacy of hazard identification and mitigation is increasingly important to morale. Command efforts to protect deployed CF elements are being complicated by such factors as the societal primacy of individual interests versus the collective good, risk misperception, barriers to the mandating of medical countermeasures, inadequate command awareness of and attention to health protection issues, and late or inadequate consideration of medical input to the planning process. Individually, some of these factors might be considered limited hindrances to effective health protection, but others have already demonstrated significant detrimental effects to individual health and operational readiness.

Societal trends in favour of greater individual rights and autonomy have helped enhance institutional regard for CF members' quality of life, morale, health, and welfare. Therefore, it is critical to health, morale, recruiting, retention, and ultimately to CF operational effectiveness that all possible measures be taken to protect CF members from health hazards. The CF's national obligation to protect society, however, often requires the performance of dangerous activities. No military can be effective if each member of the armed forces can choose which risks to accept and which to reject, since that decision may endanger the lives of others and the success of the mission. The CF's human resources strategy's "People First" focus is critically important, but its ethical principle of service to Canada before self must always prevail.[70] The focus on individual interests and welfare over the past few years is welcome and necessary, but care must be taken that the pendulum does not swing excessively to the detriment of collective and institutional interests. As in all occupational health scenarios, a reasoned balance must be struck considering individual liberties, workplace health hazards, protective countermeasures, and the occupational mission. This balance must be based on objective scientific analysis of evidence, a balanced risk assessment, and mission considerations. It must never be skewed by unsubstantiated speculation. Current societal and institutional command trends must be resisted where they may unreasonably limit the ability of commanders to apply direct and indirect health protection measures in the general unit or mission interest. The societal threats to force health protection efforts may be managed through continued command support to pre-, intra-, and post-deployment health hazard assessment and mitigation efforts, timely and widespread health risk communication efforts, and enhancements to health surveillance capabilities. Individual compliance will depend largely on the effective communication of accurate information concerning health threats and countermeasures, the development of confidence in CF command and medical authorities, and strong command support.

Inadequate command attention to or knowledge of force health protection issues has been responsible for some failures in the past, and may be in the future if awareness and responsibility are not well communicated to CF leaders. Despite significant resource allocations that have dramatically increased the CF's health protection expertise and capability, its application remains almost entirely dependant on the will, leadership, and attention of command authorities. Instead of piecemeal efforts to address knowledge gaps in prominent issues such as mental health, depleted uranium, or toxic industrial chemicals, broader training in all operationally-significant health protection issues should be an important part of all levels of command and staff training. Formal educational requirements would improve command capability competence and planning, and would ultimately contribute to greater confidence in CF leaders. Education should be progressive and appropriate to the level of responsibility, with junior leaders focusing on health threats and technical hygiene and sanitation measures, and senior leaders studying organizational, planning, policy, legal, and political health protection issues.

Operational contractor support that might affect health must be carefully planned and monitored to ensure that adequate standards are met. Contingency plans should also always be in place to permit rapid assumption of the relevant contracted duties by qualified CF personnel. Doctrinal publications should universally include preventive health measures as force protection tasks rather than uniquely as sustainment tasks. The CF should vigorously defend its authority to mandate the use of medical countermeasures, conduct realistic training, and any other measure necessary to enhance operational fitness, protect individual health, protect the force from operational hazards, and ensure mission success. Unit, formation, and mission contingent commanders should, within consistent national standards and policies, be given whatever authority and support is necessary to implement measures that directly or indirectly enhance force health protection.

Finally, history teaches us that we often do not learn from our past with respect to preventive health efforts. Although low injury and disease rates are usually the fruit of persistent and prolonged health protection and promotion efforts, their achievement is often seen as justification to scale back such programs. The reforms that have been initiated to enhance health protection in response to the report of the Croatia Board of Inquiry and other reports will not be fully implemented for years. Should the CF's current commitment to these efforts wane as recent problems recede from memory, the cycle will predictably repeat itself.

NOTES

1   H. Zinsser, *Rats, Lice and History* (Boston: Little Brown & Co., 1935), 152.

2   Zinsser, *Rats, Lice and History*, 150-165; John English, "The Operational Art: Developments in the Theories of War," in B.J.C. McKercher and Michael A. Hennessy, eds. *The Operational Art: Developments in the Theories of War* (Westport, CT: Praeger, 1996), 11; Canada, Department of National Defence (DND), Director General Health Services, *Concept for the CF Health Protection Capability* (Ottawa: DND, March 2001), 10; C.G. Cook, "Influence of Diarrhoeal Disease on Military and Naval Campaigns," *Journal of the Royal Society of Medicine* 94 (February 2001), 95-7; United States Army, *Force Health Protection in a Global Environment*, Field Manual 4-02 (Washington: Department of the Army, 2003), 1-2; Kurt A. Sanftleben, *The Unofficial Joint Medical Officers Handbook* (Bethesda, MD: Uniformed Services University of the Health Sciences, 1995), 10-11; and Arthur M. Smith, "The Influence of Medicine on Strategy," *Naval War College Review* 41, no. 2 (Spring 1988), 30.

3   DND, *Concept for the CF Health Protection Capability*, 1-2.

4   DND, *Final Report: Board of Inquiry – Croatia* (Ottawa: DND, 2000), 5; and Llewellyn J. Legters and Craig H. Llewellyn, "Military Medicine," in John Last and Robert Wallace, Cds., *Public Health & Preventive Medicine*, 13th ed. (Norwalk CT, Appleton & Lange, 1992), 1148, 1150-3.

5   DND, *Canadian Forces Operations*, B-GG-005-004/AF-000 (Ottawa: DND, 2000), p. 19-1; DND, *Final Report: Board of Inquiry – Croatia*, 26-7, 28-31, 41-3; and DND, *Concept for the CF Health Protection Capability*, 1-16.

6   Zinsser, Rats, *Lice and History*, 153.

7   M. Alice Ottoboni, *The Dose Makes the Poison: A Plain-Language Guide to Toxicology*, 2nd ed. (Indianapolis: Wiley Publishing, 1996).

8   Legters and Llewellyn, "Military Medicine," 1150, 1154; and Sanftleben, *The Unofficial Joint Medical Officers Handbook*, 1-2.

9   Zinsser, *Rats, Lice and History*, 153.

10   United States, Department of Defense (DoD), "Implement Preventive Medicine Measures," in *Medical Environmental Disease Intelligence and Countermeasures* CD-ROM (Fort Detrick: Armed Forces Medical Intelligence Center, 2001), 1.

11   Benjamin G. Withers, "Slim, Rommel, and Preventive Medicine," *Infantry* 85, no. 1 (Jan-Feb 1995), 21-2; and Ronald F. Bellamy and Craig H. Llewellyn, "Preventable Casualties: Rommel's Flaw, Slim's Edge," *Army* 40, no. 5 (May 1990), 52-5.

12   DoD, "Implement Preventive Medicine Measures," 1-4.

13   Lester W. Grau and William A. Jorgensen, "Beaten by the Bugs - The Soviet-Afghan War Experience," *Military Review* 77, no 6. (Nov-Dec 1997), 30-7.

14   DND, Canadian Forces Medical Group (CFMG) Assistant Chief of Staff Operations, *The Consequences of Ignoring Operational Medical Advice* (Ottawa: DND, 2001), 2.

15   Andy Green, "Malaria Sitrep - UK Armed Forces," presentation to Interagency Working Group for Antimalarial Chemotherapy, 16 April 2002.

16   B.K. Bohnker and S. Thornton, "Explosive Outbreaks of Gastroenteritis in the Shipboard Environment Attributed to Norovirus," *Military Medicine* 165, no. 5 (May 2003), iv; K.C. Earhart, et al., "Outbreak of Influenza in Highly Vaccinated Crew of US Navy Ship," *Emerging Infectious Diseases* 7, no. 3 (May-Jun 2001), 463-5; B.K. Bohnker, et al., "Explosive Outbreak of Gastroenteritis on an Aircraft Carrier: An Infectious Disease Mass Casualty Situation," *Aviation, Space and Environmental Medicine* 64, no. 7 (Jul 1993), 648-50; and C. Ziebold, et al., "An Outbreak of Rubella aboard a Ship of the German Navy," *Infection* 31, no. 2 (Jun 2003), 136-42.

17   United States Department of Health and Human Services, Centers for Disease Control, "Outbreak of Acute Gastroenteritis Associated with Norwalk-like Viruses among British Military Personnel - Afghanistan, May 2002," *Morbidity and Mortality Weekly* Report 51, no. 22 (7 Jun 2002), 477-9.

18   David Brown, "Malaria Outbreak Blamed on Troops," *Washington Post* (18 October 2003), A20

19   DND, *Report -Medical Theatre Assistance Visit - East Timor 13-23 February 2000* (Ottawa: DND, 29 Feb 2000).

20   DND, DCDS Group, "Operation Apollo – Lessons Learned Staff Action Directive," Annex B to 3350-165/A27, dated April 2003, pp. B-21 to B-22.

21   Major R.J.A. Tremblay, CFMG National Leader/Deployable Health Hazard Assessment Teams, personal communication, Ottawa, July 2003.

22   Author's personal experience as CFMG section head for Occupational and Environmental Health, summer 2003.

23   Lieutenant-Commander I.M. Fleming, Task Force Bosnia-Herzegovina Surgeon, E-mail to CFMG Headquarters Ottawa dated 8 Sep 2003.

24   T.H. Tulchinsky, et al., "Measles during the Gulf War: A Public Health Threat in Israel, the West Bank, and Gaza," *Public Health Review* 20, no. 3-4 (1992-93), 285-96; R.A. Gasser Jr, et al., "The Threat of Infectious Disease in Americans Returning from Operation Desert Storm," *New England Journal of Medicine* 324, no. 12 (1991), 859-64; V.L. Laurel, et al., "An Outbreak of Influenza Caused by Imported Virus in the United States, July 1999," *Clinics in Infectious Diseases* 32, no. 11 (1 Jun 2001), 1639-42; A.F. Trofa, et al., "Dengue Fever in US Military Personnel in Haiti," *Journal of the American Medical Association* 277, no. 19 (May 21 1997), 1546-8; S.C. Craig, et al., "Rubella Outbreak, Fort Bragg, North Carolina, 1995: A Clash of Two Preventive Strategies," *Military Medicine* 164, no. 9 (Sep 1999), 616-8; and J.S. Lee, et al., "Outbreak of Vivax Malaria in Areas Adjacent to the Demilitarized Zone, South Korea, 1998," *American Journal of Tropical Medicine and Hygiene* 66, no. 1 (Jan 2002), 13-17.

25   DND, *Concept for the CF Health Protection Capability*, 2-3; and DND, *Final Report: Board of Inquiry – Croatia*, 53.

26   Field Marshal William Slim, *Defeat into Victory – Battling Japan in Burma and India 1942-1945* (New York: Cooper Square Press, 2000), xi.

27   DND, *General Safety Program – General Safety Standards*, C-02-040-009/AG-001 (Ottawa: DND, 2000), chapter 1 paragraph 4.

28   DND, *Concept for the CF Health Protection Capability*, 2-3.

29   Colonel D.A. Salisbury, CFMG Deputy Chief of Staff Force Health Protection, personal communication, Ottawa, January 2003.

30   Lieutenant-Colonel Greg Cook, CFMG Director Medical Policy/Public Health, personal communication, Ottawa, June 2002.

31   DND, *Concept for the CF Health Protection Capability*, 5.

32   DND, *Concept for the CF Health Protection Capability*, 2-3; and DND, *Rx2000 Project Charter* (Ottawa: DND, 2000).

33   DND, *DCDS [Deputy Chief of the Defence Staff] Instruction 02/2000 - DCDS Direction for International Operations* (DDIO), (Ottawa: DND, 2000), Chapter 18.

34   Martin O'Malley, et al., "You and the Flu," *CBC News Backgrounder* (October 2002), available from http:www.cbc.ca/news/features/flu.html; Internet; accessed 13 October 2003.

35   Paul Vitz, *Psychology as Religion – The Cult of Self-Worship* (Grand Rapids: Eerdsmans Publishing, 1994), 84-94.

36   G.E. Sharpe and Allan D, English, "The Decade of Darkness," unpublished paper written for the CF Leadership Institute, (2003), 14; Les Perreaux, "No room for individuals in forces – commander," *Halifax Herald* (25 September 2003); and G.E. Sharpe and Allan D. English, *Principles for Change in the Post-Cold War Command and Control of the Canadian Forces*. (Kingston: Canadian Forces Leadership Institute, 2002), 57-9.

37   George Radwanski, "Privacy in Health Research: Sharing Perspectives and Paving the Way Forward," address given to the Canadian Institutes on Health Research Privacy Conference, 14 November 2002; available from http:www.privcom.gc.ca/speech/02_05_a_021114_e.asp, accessed 11 October 2003.

38   Jeff Whitehead, personal communication, January 2003.

39   US National Academy of Sciences Institute of Medicine, *Gulf War and Health: Report of the Institute of Medicine*, Carolyn Fulco, et al., eds. (Washington: National Academy of Sciences Institute of Medicine, 2000); United States, *Presidential Advisory Committee (PAC) on Gulf War Illnesses Final Report* (Washington: December 1996), 112-14, available from http:www.gwvi.ncr.gov/toc-f.html, accessed May 2001; US National Academy of Sciences Institute of Medicine, *Health Consequences of Service During the Persian Gulf War: Recommendations for Research and Information Systems* (Washington, National Academy of Sciences Institute of Medicine, 1996) 49-55, 100, available from http://books.nap.edu/books/0309055369/html/1.html, accessed May 2001; United States. "The Persian Gulf Experience and Health, National Institutes of Health Technology Assessment Workshop Panel," *Journal of the American Medical Association* 272, no. 5 (3 Aug 1994), 391-5, available from http://text.nlm.nih.gov/ftrs/tocview; and DND, *Health Study of Canadian Forces Personnel Involved in the 1991 Conflict in the Persian Gulf* (Ottawa: Goss-Gilroy Inc., 1997).

40   Slim, *Defeat into Victory*, 180.

41   Michael Gochfeld, "Toxicology," chapter 16 in Wallace and Last, eds., *Public Health & Preventive Medicine*, 324, 336; and Aerospace Medical Association, Editorial, "Protecting the Health of US Military Forces: A National Obligation," *Aviation, Space and Environmental Medicine* 71, no. 3 (March 2000), 6.

42   Ottoboni, *The Dose Makes the Poison;* Ernest Small, "Scholarly Publishing: Survive and Thrive in the Electronic Information Age," presentation at the National Research Council Press workshop, (Ottawa, 4 November 2001); and Phil Brown, "Addressing Public Distrust-Siting Hazardous Waste Treatment facilities: The NIMBY Syndrome / The Fail-Safe Society," *Technology Review* 95, no. 5 (1992), 68-70.

43   Eve Savory, "Science and Media: Bridging the Gulf," available from   http://www.publicaffairs.ubc.ca/ubcreports/1999/99mar18/99mar18for.html, accessed 10 October 2003.

44   Sharpe and English, "The Decade of Darkness," 4-6, 17-18; and Sharpe and English, *Principles for Change*, 58.

45   DND, *Canadian Forces Health and Lifestyle Information Survey* (Ottawa: DND, 2000), 7, 53; Allan D. English, "Leadership and Operational Stress in the Canadian Forces," *Canadian Military Journal* 1, no. 3 (Autumn 2000), 34; DND, *Canadian Forces Operations*, p. 19-1; G.E. Sharpe, *Croatia Board of Inquiry – Leadership (and Other) Lessons Learned* (Kingston: Canadian Forces Leadership Institute, 2002), 38; and DND, *Final Report: Board of Inquiry – Croatia,* 40.

46   Cook, personal communication; DND, *Minutes of Proceedings, Standing Court Martial, Her Majesty the Queen versus Sgt (Retired) Michael Kipling* (Ottawa: DND, 2000); and DND, "Memorandum of Fact and Law of the Appellant in the Court Martial Appeal Court of Canada Between Her Majesty The Queen and Sergeant (Retired) Michael Kipling," (Ottawa: DND, 23 October 2000).

47   C.J. Clements, "Mass Psychogenic Illness after Vaccination," *Drug Safety* 26, no. 9 (2003), 599-604; J.P. Struewing and G.C. Gray, "An Epidemic of Respiratory Complaints Exacerbated by Mass Psychogenic Illness in a Military Recruit Population," *American Journal of Epidemiology* 132, no. 6 (Dec 1990), 1120-29; C.C. Engel, Jr, "Outbreaks of Medically Unexplained Physical Symptoms after Military Action, Terrorist Threat, or Technological Disaster," *Military Medicine* 166, no. 2 Supplement (Dec 2001), 47-8; Jeff Doan, "Doctors Predict 'Hysteria' Outbreaks - Dramatic Illness at US School Blamed on Mass Anxiety," *The Ottawa Citizen* (13 January 2000); Kenneth C. Hyams, et al., "War Syndromes and Their Evaluation: From the US Civil War to the Persian Gulf War," *Annals of Internal Medicine* 125, no. 5 (1 September 1996); and United States, Agency for Toxic Substances and Disease Registry, *Report of the Expert Panel Workshop on the Psychological Responses to Hazardous Substances*, Pamela Tucker, ed. (Washington: Agency for Toxic Substances and Disease Registry, September 1995).

48   English, "Leadership and Operational Stress," 35.

49   Sharpe, *Croatia Board of Inquiry - Leadership*, 51.

50   Slim, *Defeat into Victory*, 180.

51   North Atlantic Treaty Organization (NATO), *Report of the 3rd meeting of the NATO Biological Medical*

Defence Advisory Committee, 18-19 May 1999 (The Hague: NATO, 1999).

52   Jeremy Tuck, et al., "Falciparum Malaria: An Outbreak in a Military Population on an Operational Deployment," *Military Medicine* 8, (August 2003), 639-42.

53   Stephen P. Frances, et al., "Survey of Personnel Protection Measures Against Mosquitoes Among Australian Defence Force Personnel Deployed to East Timor," *Military Medicine* 168, no. 3, (March 2003), 227-30.

54   J.A. Newton, Jr, "Malaria in US Marines Returning from Somalia," *Journal of the American Medical Association* 272, no. 5 (3 August 1994), 397-9.

55   Brown, "Malaria Outbreak," A20.

56   Salisbury, personal communication, 7 Oct 2003.

57   English, "Leadership and Operational Stress," 36; and Legters and Llewellyn, "Military Medicine,"1153.

58   Major-General Baron Silas Von Stueben, "Instructions for the Commandant of a Regiment," in *Regulations for the Order and Discipline of the Troops of the United States* (Continental Congress, 29 March 1779).

59   Ross Pigeau and Carol McCann, "Re-conceptualizing Command and Control," *Canadian Military Journal* 3, no. 1 (Spring 2002), 53-63.

60   DND, *DCDS Direction for International Operations*, 18-8, 18-9.

61   Sharpe and English, *Principles for Change*, 61-2; Sharpe and English, "The Decade of Darkness," 18-19; and DND, *Final Report: Board of Inquiry - Croatia*, 49.

62   Slim, *Defeat into Victory*, 179.

63   Susanne J. Clark, "Striking at the US Army's Strength: Soldiers - The Imperative of Biotechnology for Force Health Protection," US Army War College Strategy Research Project (Carlisle Barracks, PA: US Army War College, 7 April 2003), 16-18.

64   DND, *Canadian Forces Operations*, chapters 19, 21, 24.

65   Darryl Bradley, "Prime Vendor Support - The Wave of the Future," unpublished paper written for Canadian Forces College, Advanced Military Studies Course 5, 2000), 16-17.

66   DND, *Chief of Review Services Report on Canadian Forces Participation in the Persian Gulf War* (Ottawa: DND, 1992), 36, 40, 43, 44.

67   DND, DCDS Group, "Operation Apollo – Lessons Learned Staff Action Directive," pp. B-21, B-22.

68   Canada, *Report of the Commission of Inquiry into the Deployment of Canadian Forces to Somalia* (Ottawa: Canadian Government Publishing, 1997).

69   Author's personal experience as CFMG section head for Occupational and Environmental Health, summer 2003.

70   DND, *Military HR Strategy 2020 - Facing the People Challenges of the Future* (Ottawa: DND, 2002), 3-4.

CHAPTER 3

WHITHER THE FIELD AMBULANCE?
ROLE 2 LAND HEALTH SERVICE SUPPORT IN THE 21ST CENTURY BATTLESPACE

Colonel James C. Taylor

A well-prepared and able military medical system conveys four powerful messages. It tells the [nation's] people that its leaders have prepared means to care for their sons and daughters who may have to be sent into harm's way; it tells our adversaries that we have a credible, sustainable fighting force; it tells our military commanders that we will sustain their forces; it tells our troops that we care. The last is the most vital: in the absence of medical readiness we can have no assurance that our troops, the flesh-and-blood elements of our weapon systems, will retain the will to fight, which is the crucial factor in the equation for victory.

Rear Admiral James A. Zimble, US Navy[1]

INTRODUCTION

The requirement for the Canadian Forces (CF) capability to undertake the treatment and evacuation of casualties is set forth at the strategic, operational and tactical levels by the Vice Chief of the Defence Staff (VCDS) document *Canadian Joint Task List*.[2] Furthermore, this capability must be effective and relevant throughout the 11 CF *Force Planning Scenarios*[3] (at Annex A), which describe the challenges to be met by the CF across the spectrum of conflict.

Health Service Support (HSS) is a key element of campaign planning, and military commanders have come to rely increasingly upon medical care resources being available and capable when and where needed.[4] Moreover, HSS in theatre is ultimately the responsibility of the operational commander,[5] because, as Gouge cautions, "providing care to early casualties will be critical to mission success at the time when the medical footprint is extremely limited."[6] Indeed, modern operations can result in high casualty rates before the HSS in the theatre is fully developed. Care for early casualties may then become a key component of the success of the operation and, as such, a centre of gravity.[7] Further, in an era when nations are less and less likely to accept the possibility of casualties in support of national security, current indications are that they will not tolerate shortfalls in the provision of HSS to their deployed sons and daughters in uniform.[8]

CF HSS is based on a patient management continuum, which extends from the point of injury through successive levels of HSS capability based on patients' needs and available resources, culminating in health care facilities in Canada.[9] To enact this continuum, CF HSS is organized into Levels of Support (at Annex B), which reflect command and control relationships at each level of organization and an increasing level of sophistication of clinical capabilities; these Levels are in keeping with those expressed in NATO HSS doctrine.[10] In addition to Levels of Support, CF (and NATO) doctrine is based on progressive categories of HSS capability referred to as Roles of Health Care (at Annex C).[11]

A CF "field ambulance" is a unit-sized HSS organization that now provides Role 1 and 2 HSS to a Brigade Group at the tactical level, with ground evacuation from Role 1 elements. Informal and formal debate[12] has taken place as to whether, with the establishment of the "hub and spoke" model of tactical air evacuation (which is based on the concept of air evacuation of patients directly from Role 1 to Role 3),[13] the current-ly-configured field ambulance would no longer be relevant and that forward surgical capability and rotary-wing aeromedical evacuation (AME) would become the norm. It will be argued here that this idea is both correct and incorrect, and that the capability resident within an evolved Role 2 HSS organization is an essential element of the CF patient management continuum if we are to meet the exigencies of providing HSS that is relevant to all force planning scenarios.

A precept of CF HSS doctrine is that "health care shall be provided at all levels of accessibility and quality comparable to those being afforded to the Canadian public generally."[14] This capability has been benchmarked to the clinical capability available in a Canadian Level 2 (District) Trauma Centre.[15] NATO doctrine on standards of care states that:

Medical support to NATO forces must meet standards acceptable to all participating nations. Even in crisis or conflict, the aim is to provide a standard of medical care as close as possible to prevailing peacetime national medical standards, given the difficulties of doing so in an operational setting. Advances in medical and information technologies should be exploited to keep the operational standard of care as close as possible to peacetime standards and to deliver emergency care and emergency surgery as close as possible to the point of wounding.[16]

It then goes on to require that units and formations engaged in NATO operations deploy and re-deploy with a coherent medical structure.[17] This paper will discuss that coherent medical structure, in a format intended for a general military readership and focusing on Role 2 capabilities, in the context of clinical concepts, allied doctrine and the history of military HSS.

THE GOLDEN HOUR

The term "Golden Hour" was coined in the early 1970s to express the idea that the first hour following injury is when definitive care is critical to a trauma patient's survival.[18] Although the specifics and supporting data for this concept continue to undergo debate,[19] it is accepted as a benchmark in current trauma management,[20] and is directly referenced in CF HSS and NATO Joint Medical Support doctrine.[21] The American College of Surgeons, which publishes the widely-used Advanced Trauma Life Support (ATLS) protocols, describes the Golden Hour or "first hour" of care following injury as being "characterized by the need for rapid assessment and resuscitation."[22]

Besides the "Golden Hour," the Tri-modal Distribution of Casualty Death is another useful model for examining a trauma patient's survival. In this model, casualty deaths peak at three points: the first peak at seconds to minutes for severely injured patients, the second peak at minutes to hours for patients with significant blood loss, and the third peak at hours to days, usually due to sepsis (infection) and multiple organ failure.[23] This distribution is illustrated graphically at Figure 3-1.[24]

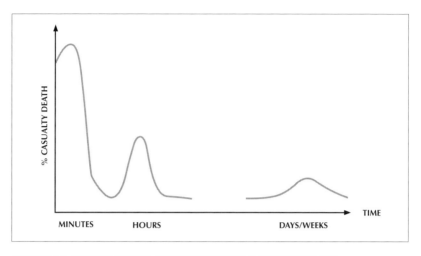

FIGURE 3-1 THE TRI-MODAL DISTRIBUTION OF CASUALTY DEATH.

In military medicine, combat mortality is divided into two categories: 1) casualties that die prior to entry into the HSS system and are classified as KIA (Killed in Action), and 2) casualties who die after having entered the HSS system and are classified as DOW (Died of Wounds).[25] Smith reports that "estimates indicate that nearly 20 percent of those who die during combat suffer from surgically correctable injuries and might have been saved except for delays in the application of definitive treatment."[26] The importance of time in the treatment of battle casualties was known as early as the First World War. Military physicians recognized at that time that if the badly wounded patient who reached a treatment facility was given adequate shock therapy within one hour of being wounded, his chances of survival were 90 percent, as opposed to 25 percent after eight hours.[27] A recent US study comparing civilian rural pre-hospital care of major trauma reported that victims were 7.4 times as likely to die before arrival if the emergency medical services' response time was more than 30 minutes.[28]

CF and NATO HSS doctrine emphasizes time, specifically that period of time which elapses between injury and the initiation of definitive treatment, as being a key factor in the morbidity and mortality (death an disability) of patients, and that resuscitation and stabilization should be undertaken within the first hour following injury. It distinguishes, however, between life/limb-saving surgery and that which must take place to remove contaminated tissue (debridement), which could otherwise result in a life-threatening infection within six hours. Hence, the doctrinal guideline for time to intervention is: "Life/limb-saving clinical interventions must be provided as soon as possible, ideally within the first hour, but completed not later than six hours following onset of life/limb-threatening injury."[29] However, the traditional first level of HSS where a "life/limb-saving surgery" capability exists is at the Role 3 field hospital. Thus, the solutions to the time-to-initial-surgery challenge have been focused on the movement of a surgical capability forward to the patient and/or the acceleration of the movement of the patient to the surgical capability via forward AME.

FORWARD SURGICAL CAPABILITY

HSS facilities are doctrinally located "as far forward as possible without interfering with operations or unnecessarily subjecting patients to hostile action," with the positioning of resources such that initial surgery can be undertaken as rapidly as possible.[30] For example, during the Inchon landing in Korea in 1950, the effectiveness of the medical battalion supporting the US 1st Marine Division landing force was significantly enhanced by moving advanced surgical teams forward to the clearing-unit level (Role 2).[31] During the 1970s, the Israeli Defence Force (IDF) deployed forward surgical trauma teams able to resuscitate and stabilize casualties who could not immediately be moved to field hospitals.[32] The IDF established a mini-combat-trauma centre on the Sinai front to which the seriously wounded were sent to prior to their evacuation to Israeli hospitals far to the rear. In deciding whether to operate, the patients' clinical condition was weighed against the estimated rigours of a long evacuation.[33] In the final years of the Soviet conflict in Afghanistan, by moving special surgical teams close to the fighting in preparation for planned large offensive operations, the Soviets reduced their DOW rate of the moderately wounded from 4.3 percent to 2 percent.[34] NATO HSS doctrine notes that a certain cohort among casualties will require forward emergency surgery as soon as possible following injury to minimize morbidity and mortality and that when necessary, this surgery renders the casualty transportable to a higher level of HSS for definitive care.[35] CF doctrine describes initial surgery as "resuscitative and stabilizing surgical intervention that must be performed urgently and as far forward as the tactical situation permits, in order to save life and limb, and control hemorrhage and infection."[36]

The HSS doctrinal documents of all four US services mandate a surgical capability, either integral or by augmentation, in their Role 2 elements. The US Army Echelon 2 (Roles are referred to as Echelons in US HSS doctrine) organization is the Forward Medical Support Company, which on its own is clinically a Role 2 capability but may be augmented to a Role 2+ capability with the attachment of a Forward Surgical Team to provide a resuscitative surgery capability.[37] The US Air Force Echelon 2 organization is the Air Transportable Clinic that supports the Squadron Medical Element; this HSS asset has a Role 2 capability and can be augmented to a Role 2+ or greater capability with the progressive modular deployment of elements of the US Air Force EMEDS (Expeditionary Medical Support) System.[38] In the US Navy, the Echelon 2 HSS capability resides aboard the aircraft carrier of a Carrier Battle Group and the Casualty Receiving Treatment Ships of an Amphibious Battle Group, and it has a baseline Role 2+ capability with integral resuscitative surgical capability.[39] The US Marine Corps Echelon 2 organization is the Medical Battalion, which has a baseline Role 2+ capability. Its resuscitative surgical capability resides within the Surgical Platoons of its three surgical companies and its eight Shock Trauma Platoons.[40] The Commander-in-Chief of US Central Command from 1994-97 summarized US forward surgical capability doctrine this way: "When casualties occur the battlefield will be cleared. Patients will be stabilized forward with light surgical teams then moved rearward, maintaining en route care and accountability."[41]

The Canadian Forces Health Services (CFHS) has undertaken a major phased review of CF HSS deployable clinical capabilities through its Standing Committee on Operational Medicine Review (SCOMR). At the tactical level, the Committee recommended that forward HSS be provided by a close support composite Role 2+ unit, i.e., a Role 2 unit with integral Role 1 and augmentable with a surgical capability.[42] The most recent CF HSS doctrine reflects augmentation of Role 2 with a clinical surgical capability module that is provided by the Role 3 HSS units, with such modular augmentation being undertaken in multiples if a continuous 24/7 capability is required. This module comprises a team of five to seven personnel along with all basic equipment necessary to provide surgical care, and is the basic platform for the addition of sub-specialty modules.[43] Elements ranging from a field surgical team to an advanced surgical centre may be attached.[44]

Future combat will likely be at a greater pace with a greater degree of dispersal of supported units, increasing the value of highly mobile HSS treatment assets. The increased range and accuracy of weapons, combined with the possible lack of compunction of future adversaries regarding the targeting of HSS facilities, will make a potential target of the larger-footprint lower-mobility Role 3 organizations for which rear areas were traditionally a relative sanctuary.[45] The traditional Role 2 field ambulance is a highly mobile HSS asset; it must be recognized, however, that with the benefit of increasing capability through modular augmentation comes an increased requirement for HSS personnel and materiel, and a consequent reduction in mobility.[46] The added value to the task-tailored modular augmentation of the evolved Role 2 HSS capability is that a flexible balance can be made, and adjusted as required, between clinical capability and tactical mobility for dynamic operational circumstances. Enhanced treatment capabilities notwithstanding, the historic and ongoing role of the field ambulance as a key element of Forward Medical Evacuation bears further exploration. US Air Force physicians assigned to the United Nations Protection Force in the former Yugoslavia (UNPROFOR), where Field Surgical Teams (FSTs) were deployed forward to augment Role 1, observed that FSTs partially "compensated for the deficiencies (in evacuation), but do not replace the need for Medical Evacuation"; however, they also advised that "a good Medical Evacuation capability will complement the FSTs but never replace them."[47]

HISTORY OF MILITARY CASUALTY EVACUATION

The rapid casualty evacuation system has been an integral part of military HSS during major conflicts since its development in 1795 by Baron Dominique Jean Larrey, a French surgeon during the Napoleonic Wars. Napoleon ensured that each of his divisions had an ambulance corps comprising 170 men, a surgeon and purpose-built horse-drawn carriages to carry casualties to the rear for rapid surgical intervention. In 1862, Major Jonathan Letterman, Medical Director of the Army of the Potomac during the US Civil War, implemented a hierarchical evacuation system whereby ambulances would bring all casualties as quickly as possible to a clearing station immediately to the rear of each battlefront, where they were sorted. Seriously wounded patients underwent lifesaving surgery as soon as possible, and then were transported to hospitals in the rear. Lightly wounded patients were treated later and kept near the front lines.

The foundation of the current echelon care system was implemented by the Allies during the First World War: First Aid Stations (Role 1) located behind Regimental Reserves for rapid initial treatment (including basic surgery); Ambulance Squads (approximately Role 2 less clinical care) to then transport rearward patients who required further care; Field Hospitals (Role 3), located behind Divisional Reserves, for urgent surgery, followed by railway evacuation rearward of patients who could not return to duty; civilian Hospitals (approximating Role 4), for convalescence and further care as required.[48]

The first reported air evacuation is generally thought to have occurred during the siege of Paris in 1870 during the Franco-Prussian War, where 160 casualties were evacuated by balloon.[49] The first fixed-wing tactical evacuation was performed during the First World War by the French from the Albanian Front in 1915 in an aircraft of opportunity; an aerial ambulance service using purpose-modified aircraft to evacuate combat casualties was initiated by the French in April 1918 in Flanders.[50] The first rotary-wing combat air evacuation mission was flown in Burma (today also called Myanmar) in April 1944 by the US Army Air Forces, with a number of further instances recorded in 1944-45 in the Pacific Theatre.[51] Korea saw helicopter air evacuation become an established practice, with US Army helicopter ambulance detachments assigned to Mobile Army Surgical Hospitals (MASH) for the rapid evacuation of seriously-injured soldiers from the front line to the appropriate level of medical treatment. Over 17,000 Allied casualties were evacuated by air evacuation during the Korean War.[52] Helicopter tactical air evacuation evolved significantly in the Vietnam War, and was responsible for the evacuation of nearly 900,000 Allied sick and wounded; also of import is the fact that in Vietnam, most combat units were within a half hour's flight from a Role 3 or Role 4 facility.[53] Although it must be borne in mind that there were significant advances in medical science and techniques between the First World War and the Vietnam War, the concurrent improvements in casualty evacuation certainly contributed to the decreasing US DOW rates: 8.5 percent in the First World War, 4 percent in the Second World War, 2 percent in Korea, and 1 percent in Vietnam.[54]

With the evolution of patient evacuation has come the evolution of differential terminology to describe it. CASEVAC (Casualty Evacuation) pertains to patient transport from the site of injury to a medical treatment facility using generic transport (e.g., "lift of opportunity") without the provision of substantive en route medical care, and represents the "scoop and run" method employed in mass casualty situations. True MEDEVAC (Medical Evacuation) resembles the civilian medical transport model (including AME and ground MEDEVAC [GME]), with appropriately trained and equipped personnel providing en route medical care.[55]

FORWARD AEROMEDICAL EVACUATION

The clinical requirement for universal civilian AME is still debated in the literature. Seven studies have been undertaken in various regions of the US comparing mortality rates for trauma patients transported by rotary-wing AME versus GME. Four reported that mortality rates were decreased for patients transported by helicopter,[56] while three reported no difference in mortality rates.[57] It must be recognized, however, that these studies were undertaken in the context of an intact civilian infrastructure in peacetime.

CF doctrine defines Forward AME as providing airlift for patients within areas of tactical level operations, usually with tactical aviation resources. It has the advantages of speed, range, comfort and flexibility of destination facility. The CF doctrinal HSS staffing for Forward AME normally comprises one Medical Assistant Primary Care Paramedical (Enhanced Skills certified), provided by the field ambulance,[58] and is in harmony with SCOMR clinical recommendations.[59] NATO doctrine states that Forward AME is normally a national responsibility, and that AME aircraft must be medically equipped and crewed in line with the minimum requirements of the applicable NATO standing agreement (STANAG 3204 *Aeromedical Evacuation*) and national standards.[60]

As we have seen, a precept of CF HSS doctrine is that "health care shall be provided at all levels of accessibility and quality comparable to those being afforded to the Canadian public generally."[61] The vast majority of the Canadian populace has access to rotary-wing AME for rapid transport (with in-flight sustaining care by a certified EMT-Paramedic) to a District Trauma Centre or higher medical facility. The key elements of this service are: a dedicated pre-configured helicopter, dedicated and appropriately-qualified personnel on standby, and dedicated communication lines.[62] The Alberta STARS (Shock Trauma Air Rescue Society) AME crew comprises at a minimum one critical care nurse and one critical care paramedic, with the capability to augment with an ER physician or specialty teams as required. The Québec ÉVAQ (*Évacuations Aéromédicales du Québec*) medical teams are composed of physicians and ER nurses. The Ontario Air Ambulance Service flight medical teams include critical care and advanced care paramedics.[63] The medical aircrew component of the standard US Army air ambulance company MEDEVAC helicopter consists of a flight medical aidmen (flight medic), who is responsible for providing patient assessment and in-flight medical care. However, Gerhardt (a US Army Medical Officer) asserted that "in terms of our own [US Army] definitions, official doctrine, and training standards, we are in fact providing a service that is closer to CASEVAC, rather than MEDEVAC," and recommended that the medical aircrew member be instead an EMT-Paramedic.[64]

US Army doctrine describes *dedicated* MEDEVAC systems (the more preferred option), whereby the aircraft is solely dedicated/ equipped/ manned for the mission of aeromedical evacuation, in contrast to *lift of opportunity systems* (the less preferred option), whereby empty aircraft are used for CASEVAC during the backhaul following the completion of their primary mission.[65] Bauer, a US Navy Medical Officer who served with the US Marine Corps during the first Gulf War, stated that "opportune lift is a random, unpracticed participant in what has to be an organized yet highly flexible system." He recalled a US Marine Corps pilot during the first Gulf War, who had observed that "it makes no sense for us to risk our necks just to have the guy die en route."[66] Despite the fact that more than 33,000 medical personnel were deployed in Operation Desert Storm, including at least 3,100 physicians in the Gulf theatre of operations, the US Navy Surgeon General noted that "the lack of dedicated tactical aeromedical evacuation capability in naval services would have created difficulties had the theater (Southwest Asia) matured as expected."[67] A US General Accounting Office report concluded that the Army would not have been able to provide adequate care if the ground war had started sooner, lasted longer, or if casualty numbers (458 wounded) had matched casualty estimates (20,000+).[68]

The US Army has integral air ambulance units that are freestanding company- or platoon-sized elements commanded by a Medical Service Corps aviation officer (pilot). The standard company is composed of 15 UH-60

(Blackhawk) air ambulances and their associated aircrew.[69] Each Air Ambulance Evacuation Platoon has three Forward Support MEDEVAC Teams of three UH-60s who provide MEDEVAC from the point of injury or Role 1 facility to higher levels of clinical care.[70] The US Marine Corps has no integral dedicated tactical air ambulance units; US Marine Corps rotary wing transport and utility aircraft are allocated to perform the Forward AME mission at the discretion of the line commander.[71] The US Navy also has no organic capability for forward AME.[72] Smith notes that the distances involved in littoral manoeuvre, as well as its inherent limitations in GME and forward casualty treatment capability, combined with the vulnerability of units ashore, indicate a requirement for dedicated AME for this type of operation.[73]

In CF doctrine, none of the HSS units or formations has integral AME aircraft, and any AME must be coordinated by the HSS unit with the assistance of their air liaison officer.[74] All CF aircraft used in AME are "aircraft of opportunity" with no dedicated flight time for AME. Forward AME is primarily undertaken using the CH-146 Griffin in support of the Army.[75] SCOMR remarked on a current HSS capability shortfall in this regard and recommended that a number of CF CH-146 Griffin helicopters (or other purpose-procured rotary-wing aircraft) be designated to meet these key requirements in order to provide a dedicated CF MEDEVAC capability.[76] Given the lessons learned by our Allies in recent conflicts, and the CF mandate to provide a deployed health care capability comparable to that being afforded to the Canadian public generally, the CF would be wise to give close consideration to this issue.

Although dedicated Forward AME is an essential element of an effective deployed HSS capability, it does have limitations. CF doctrine describes the disadvantages of Forward AME as including physiologic stress on certain categories of patients, susceptibility to inclement weather, lack of available air space and/or AME assets as a result of enemy or friendly actions, the resource-intense nature of air operations (especially in the case of rotary-wing aircraft), the compromise of security caused by the presence of aircraft, and the tendency to evacuate patients further rearward than necessary.[77] Several of these limitations will be discussed next.

Patient Stress. A number of clinical criteria that preclude AME due to patient stress are described in NATO STANAG 3204. Further

unfavourable clinical ramifications of rotary-wing AME are also identified, including vibration (causing resonance of damaged body structures)
and turbulence (causing motion sickness), as well as noise and space/light
limitations, which complicate en route care.[78]

Weather. While there are myriad examples that could be provided of
inclement weather hindering AME, one that will be in recent memory of
many is that of the Balkans.   Although rotary-wing flying limits for
Operation Palladium (NATO Stabilization Force December 1995 -
December 2004) rotations have used 500/1 (500-foot ceiling, 1 mile visibility), as a planning figure, weather limits for wartime operational flying
(including Forward AME) would be 300/1.[79] The following table shows
the number of days by month in Velika Kladusa (VK) where conditions
fell below 300/1 during the period indicated in Figure 3-2.[80]

Sep01	Oct01	Nov01	Dec01	Jan02	Feb02	Mar02	Apr02	May02	Jun02	Jul02	Aug02
08	15	06	04	05	04	04	08	09	03	03	10

FIGURE 3-2: DAYS BELOW 300/1 IN VK BETWEEN SEP 2001 AND AUG 2002.

Similarly, US Air Force medical officers reported that weather was a significant factor for AME during their tour on UNPROFOR from October
1993 to September 1994.[81] And Krekorian described situations in
Vietnam where adverse weather precluded AME, upon which an installa-
tion was entirely reliant, leaving the Battalion Surgeon (General Duty
Medical Officer at Role 1 HSS) to provide whatever emergency surgical
care he could, with mixed clinical outcomes.[82]

Lack of Dedicated AME Aircraft. Beyond the previous discussion of the
perils of using CASEVAC lift of opportunity versus dedicated MEDEVAC,
excerpts from two published accounts from the first Gulf War will serve
to further illustrate this point. Davis, a US Marine Corps officer, described
the dilemma this way:

> The Marine Corps has only a limited number of assault support
> helicopters to undertake all the missions assigned...As this fleet
> of helicopters dwindles, mission priorities are set and (CASE-
> VACS) do not always get top billing.   Herein lies the Corps'
> dilemma: what has more importance on the battlefield – an
> assault support helicopter or a Marine's life and limb? To many

of us there does not appear to be a choice at all. Life is paramount. This is definitely true in peacetime, but what about wartime? The helicopters assigned as (CASEVACS) cannot help the group commander who needs trooplift support for his counterattack force. They also cannot be employed for an ammo resupply mission…This is a hard question that most combat commanders will eventually have to answer.[83]

Bauer, a US Navy Flight Surgeon, described his experience with having only lift of opportunity as follows:

There are no assurances that lift helos would be in the vicinity or tactically available for the [CASEVAC] of the wounded. Similarly, there would be conflicts or confusion if patient delivery points were not tactically convenient, and there would always be the risk that the helo could be suddenly diverted to a more 'critical' mission.[84]

Smith warns further that in future conflicts, "the finite number of helicopters on hand, many will be unavailable because of tactical missions, bad weather, or technical constraints."[85]

Vulnerability to Enemy Fire. Historically, rotary wing military aircraft have encountered periods of significant misfortune during times of conflict. In Vietnam, despite a negligible air-to-air threat, the US Army lost an estimated 5,086 helicopters.[86] In the first 18 months of the Soviet occupation of Afghanistan, mujahedin ground-based antiaircraft fire reportedly led to the loss of 250 Soviet helicopters. And during the 10-week Falklands War the Royal Navy lost more than 20 helicopters.[87] During the 1983 US invasion of Grenada, seven US H-60 Blackhawk and two AH-1 Cobra helicopters were lost, which represented over 10 percent of the 88 combat helicopters deployed on this operation.[88] Based on these experiences, projected combat attrition for US UH-60s in a conventional war scenario would far outstrip the industrial production capacity required to replace them, leaving this airframe in deficit for approximately 4.5 years from the initiation of conflict.[89] Consequently, Smith suggests that "assumptions that place heavy reliance upon evacuation of the wounded by helicopter or the MV-22 Osprey tilt-wing aircraft may well require reexamination."[90]

Numerous authors have recognized the clinical successes of casualty management in Vietnam that were attributable to rapid AME from point of wounding to a Role 3 or 4 treatment capability; they also maintain, however, that is was a phenomenon that will be irreproducible in future conflicts.[91] Smith described the Vietnam situation as an "aberration," which "approached the civilian concept of emergency care more closely than any war we had in the past, or are likely to have in the future."[92] Kitfield argued that from a medical support perspective, the Vietnam conflict was unique and represented "the golden age of military medicine" which is not likely to be duplicated.[93] Eiseman described the Vietnam medical support experience as the "halcyon days of American military medicine," and contends that "control of the Vietnamese battlefield, which made rapid patient evacuation a reality, was based upon several factors: command of the air and sea; fire superiority; uninterrupted radio communications; episodic battle; plenty of helicopters; relatively low casualty levels; and an enemy that lacked shoulder-mounted homing missile-type weapons."[94] For example, Stewart noted that: "We would literally stop the war [in Vietnam], bring the helicopter in and pick up [casualties], take them away and start shooting again. We owned the air and could do as we pleased most of the time."[95]

Many[96] who have made projections about the role of helicopter-based forward AME in future conflicts note that because "the quality and simplicity of small, shoulder-mounted homing missile-type weapons has increased greatly,"[97] that "the modern battlefield may be too lethal for evacuation of the wounded exclusively by air" as "the survivability of helicopters is certainly not assured."[98] Smith goes on to make the somewhat gloomy prediction that "instead of medical extractions in minutes, we may have to return to the hand litter, wheeled vehicles, or 'walking' casualties."[99] Therefore, Dorland, a former US Army AME pilot in Vietnam, suggests that the primitive evacuation methods used in the US Civil War still merit consideration on the battlefield of the future.[100]

Besides the increased threat from small surface-to-air missiles, Allied air superiority may also become increasingly difficult to guarantee. This lack of air superiority will further hamper AME[101] and could lead to increased mortality rates similar to those reported by the British during the Falklands War.[102] A number of commentators have expressed concern that because of US dependence on aeromedical evacuation, US forces do not have an adequate ground evacuation capability.[103] An example of this shortfall in dedicated Forward GME has been described in detail for the US Marine Corps during the first Gulf War.[104]

However, NATO doctrine states "to achieve its mission, a medical evacuation system must have…the ability to evacuate casualties to a medical facility 24 hours a day, in all weather, over all terrain and in any operational scenario." Hence, an enhanced GME capability, the historic purview of the field ambulance, must be maintained in accordance with other NATO doctrine which states "ground transport evacuation means should always be planned to cover all situations where AME is not possible due to operational or geographic/climatic factors."[105]

FORWARD GROUND MEDICAL EVACUATION

According to CF doctrine, the responsibility for patient evacuation is from rear to front, with supporting HSS Units relieving supported HSS Units of their patients.[106] A significant integral dedicated GME capability is inherent in both the historical and the evolved Role 1+2 field ambulance, and meets this doctrinal requirement to evacuate patients from point of injury to Role 1 and Role 2 facilities. We have seen why some have recommended less reliance on AME, particularly rotary-winged AME, and advocated improved ground ambulance capability. Hammick speculates that "the bulk of movement in forward areas is likely to remain vehicular – either tracked or wheeled – and for maintenance reasons, these will have to retain commonality with the rest of the fighting-vehicle fleet." He goes on to suggest that while combatants *may* respect the Red Cross/Crescent on military treatment facilities, as was the case in the Egyptian-Israeli conflict in the Negev in 1973, "this would not necessarily apply to the evacuation system which would still have to run the gauntlet of enemy interdiction, particularly at the forward edge of the battlefield."[107] Indeed, reports on HSS during the Russian assault on Grozny indicate that the Chechen fighters respected neither military treatment facilities nor the evacuation system, which likely came as somewhat of a surprise to most of the world's populace in the closing years of the 20th century. It was reported that the Chechens attacked and destroyed a Russian field hospital,[108] and deliberately targeted Russian medical units and evacuation helicopters. Therefore, the Russians often had to delay medical evacuation until nightfall, and rely on ground evacuation.[109] Grau and Thomas describe the Russian evacuation system:

> Wounded were normally evacuated to the regimental medical post by makeshift armored ambulances (BTR-80), since the Chechens fired on the soft-sided ambulances. Forward air evacuation was not used much, particularly after the Chechens shot down several MEDEVAC helicopters. The fighting in Grozny proved the need for a specially-designed armored ambulance.[110]

Hence, while there is a need for state-of-the-art soft-skinned ambulances to conduct the bulk of the GME activity in the forward area overall,[111] there is also a specific requirement for an armoured ambulance capability, as described in NATO doctrine: "In forward areas, armour-protected ambulances are used to afford some degree of protection for casualties and medical personnel."[112]

SCOMR remarked that the standard LSVW wheeled ambulance, while capable in many deployed tactical scenarios, was not sufficiently durable for the extremes of tactical field operations, and recommended that the armoured Bison ambulance variant be considered as the standard field ambulance for forward GME operations. Clinical staffing of the armoured Bison ambulance would comprise one Advanced Care Paramedic and one Primary Care Paramedic, similar to the AME staffing recommendation discussed previously.[113] Armoured ambulances are currently part of CF HSS doctrine[114] for use in forward areas, and are currently deployed on OP PALLADIUM (Balkans) and OP APOLLO (Southwest Asia) integral to Role 1 HSS elements.[115] When the paper on which this chapter was based was written in the fall of 2002, 23 Bison Wheeled Light Armoured Vehicles had been re-roled as ambulances;[116] and 51 were scheduled to be fielded in 2003/2004. In total, 66 were scheduled to be distributed to the restructured Role 1+2 field ambulances.[117] According to CF doctrine, HSS staffing of the armoured Bison ambulance should comprise one Medical Assistant Primary Care Paramedical (Enhanced Skills certified) and one Medical Assistant Primary Care Paramedical certified.[118] It should be noted that while a large number of nations have chosen ambulance variants of their main wheeled armoured fighting vehicles to satisfy the requirements of speed, mobility and protection,[119] others have chosen purpose-built soft-skinned vehicles because they offer more space and are more readily identifiable as ambulances by enemy forces.[120]

CONTINUITY OF CARE

> If appropriate priority is not given to forward medical care, evacuation, and a sophisticated casualty regulation network, a commander runs the risk of a huge logistical burden and an adverse impact on morale as the dead and injured accumulate. Inattention to these issues will mean the loss of trained troops who could have been treated, stabilized, and even returned to duty.[121]
>
> Captain Arthur M. Smith, US Naval Reserve (retired)

Beyond its treatment, evacuation and mobility capabilities described previously, the field ambulance has the essential HSS capability of patient sorting, staging, and holding. It should be noted that the holding function of a Role 2(+) field ambulance is significantly more limited, in both volume and duration, than that of a Role 3 facility. It is, however, a valuable forward "capacitance" capability during periods of interrupted evacuation.[122] Although these are not necessarily concepts that would commonly be incorporated to a great extent in Canadian civilian trauma management, Canada's deployed HSS requirements for warfighting should better reflect the caveat of Smith and Bellamy that "war surgery is not synonymous with civilian trauma management."[123]

CF doctrine on continuity of care mirrors that of NATO and requires that "treatment must be continuous and progressive to the level necessary for definitive treatment of patients' conditions to minimize mortality and morbidity."[124] It further states that patients should be evacuated through a series of HSS facilities, each with an increasing capability for treatment (i.e., Role 1 to Role 2 to Role 3, etc.), and that "sorting of patients to reflect priorities for treatment and evacuation or return to duty shall be conducted at every HSS treatment facility."[125] US Army doctrine states that, "routinely bypassing an echelon of care will not be practiced."[126] British joint doctrine recognizes that even for Operations Other Than War (OOTW), initial insertion of a force may not be into a benign environment, and that "conventional echeloning of medical assets may therefore be required for force protection reasons and to avoid obstructing military activity" until an area has been "stabilized and dominated by force."[127]

Evacuation doctrine allows for patient-care flexibility at the tactical level, so that HSS resources can respond to rapidly evolving tactical and/or operational scenarios. This doctrine ensures that while the minor sick and injured are treated and returned to duty as far forward as reasonable, the seriously ill or wounded are evacuated to appropriate treatment as rapidly as possible.[128] Basic US Marine Corps/US Navy doctrine requires that no patient be evacuated further to the rear than his or her medical condition requires or the military situation demands.[129] Historically, from the Second World War through to the Vietnam War, this practice has resulted in the following outcomes: 30-40 percent of wounded Marines were treated at Role 2, about 25 percent were treated at Role 3, and 37 percent were transferred out of theatre.[130] Smith and Llewellyn summarize the importance of the principle of the "hub and spoke" medical evacuation paradigm for OOTW as follows: "when the field medical system is functioning efficiently, it should be able to 'fix forward' to prevent itself from becoming a giant evacuation conduit through which trained, experienced soldiers and marines pour out of the theater to rear-echelon health care facilities."[131]

CF doctrine holds that Forward AME should be used whenever possible to transport seriously injured/ill patients from as close as practical to their point of injury/illness to a Role 3 facility (as per the Vietnam experience).[132] NATO, US Joint, British Joint, and CF doctrine espouse, if not in name then conceptually, the "hub and spoke" medical evacuation paradigm, as shown in Figure 3-3, for OOTW on a mission-dependant basis.[133] This model is described in NATO terms as "the Role 3 (HSS facility) placed centrally, with the sending units [undefined, but presumably Roles 1 and 2] arranged around it." According to British doctrine, in the "hub and spoke" model Role 2 assets are used "to reinforce the primary care matrix."[134] Powell raised concerns about patient evacuation on the more extended and dispersed future battlefield, stating that the concomitantly extended patient transit times will necessitate stabilization of injuries nearer to the point of injury prior to transport.[135] Further, as previously discussed, CF doctrine states that the benefit for the patient of immediate transfer to a Role 3 facility must be weighed against the patient's condition and the patient's consequent ability or inability to withstand the environmental rigours of the transit.[136] This practice also, of course, assumes a tactically permissive environment. Hooton has predicted that "uninhibited aeromedical evacuation of casualties from the front to the rear area hospital may not be able to occur in the future."[137] And Mullen reminds us that "operational constraints may dictate that evacuation cannot be accomplished at all."[138]

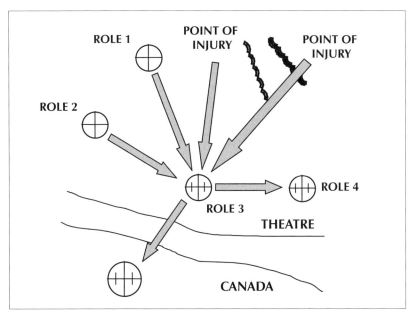

FIGURE 3-3: CF SCHEMATIC OF THE HUB-AND-SPOKE CONCEPT.

CF doctrine also recognizes that the direct Role 1 to Role 3 AME capability may be subject to interruption for a variety of reasons, necessitating evacuation of these seriously injured patients via a Role 2 facility to a surgical capability (i.e., Role 2+ or higher) as an acceptable alternative.[139] Beyond the patient holding requirement that this would precipitate, it should be remembered that the concomitant sustaining care may be provided at the unaugmented Role 2 facility, with the additional capability of resuscitative and stabilizing initial surgical intervention at the Role 2+ augmented field ambulance.[140] Liston has warned that although Bosnia has been a success in bringing a North American civilian standard of care to deployed personnel, few would dispute the impracticality of attempting to apply the HSS experience of Bosnia to a future major conventional conflict.[141]

CONCLUSION

The CF must have a deployable HSS capability for treatment and evacuation that is valid across the eleven Force Planning Scenarios. Further, this capability must meet the expectation of the Canadian populace that it can provide a Canadian standard of care to our deployed personnel, while, in the interest of interoperability, conforming to Allied doctrine to the greatest extent possible.

The continuing relevance of the traditional CF Role 2 field ambulance has been questioned in recent years, as the majority of CF deployments during that time have been on operations other than war and these operations have permitted the use of the hub-and-spoke model of medical evacuation and treatment, which is the military HSS posture that most closely resembles the civilian paradigm of care available to the majority of people in Canada. This military HSS model involves the direct aeromedical evacuation of patients to a Role 3 HSS facility, and bypasses the traditional echeloning of patient evacuation and care. While this approach has enjoyed successes in certain conflicts, including the Vietnam War and many periods during the last decade of peace support operations, history and doctrine recognize that it requires a tactically permissive environment, and it may not be sufficiently resilient to either significant increases in volume of casualties or to diminution of elements of its significant resource requirements.

The echeloned system of deployed military care has its roots in the Napoleonic Wars and the US Civil War, and is based on the requirement to provide the necessary clinical intervention as close as possible to the point of injury, in both time and space, within the constraints of the tactical situation. It embodies the concept of rapid initial lifesaving clinical care and onward evacuation of more-seriously injured patients, and the forward treatment and return to duty of less-seriously injured patients. The intent of Canadian HSS to provide a deployed standard of care benchmarked to that generally available in the national civilian health care system, superimposed on the requirement for the preservation in-theatre of scarce and highly-trained military human resources for the commander, oblige the CF to possess a robust system of forward clinical intervention and evacuation capabilities.

Detailed reports and recommendations from experiences in recent conflicts, as well as the analyses and predictions of military scholars, have
given a strong indication of the elements of HSS capability that will be
necessary in order to provide effective HSS in the predicted environment
of increased lethality of future conflicts. The benefits of dedicated
rotary-wing aeromedical evacuation assets, staffed with appropriately
qualified personnel, have been recognized, as have the intrinsic shortfalls
of systems relying on unstaffed "lifts of opportunity." While dedicated
aeromedical evacuation is an essential capability, the hazards of
over-reliance on this mode of evacuation have been identified in the
context of its dependence on weather, tactical availability of airspace,
positional security compromise, and resource intensiveness. Hence, there
remains a requirement for an in-depth ground medical evacuation
capability, the historic purview of Role 2 HSS organizations, comprising
purpose-modified armoured and soft-skinned vehicles.

Military HSS experience in previous conflicts, combined with current
civilian clinical literature and protocols, has indicated the importance of
rapid initial surgical intervention in the clinical management of severe
trauma in order to reduce patient morbidity and mortality. The Allied
doctrinal HSS embodiment of this clinical reality is the forward surgical
capability, whereby HSS Role 2 organizations have either an organic or
augmented capability to provide initial lifesaving surgery. Along with
this surgical capability, there is a requirement for limited forward patient
holding and sustaining care capabilities, organic to Role 2 HSS organizations, when clinical, tactical or logistic factors prevent the further
evacuation of patients to Role 3 or higher facilities.

Ongoing phased studies of the CF HSS capabilities necessary to meet
CF requirements have been undertaken and have identified capability
elements that have been incorporated into current CF HSS doctrine. This
doctrine now includes an evolved field ambulance with organic Role 1
and 2 assets, modularly augmentable to Role 2+ with a surgical
capability. Armoured ambulances and enhanced soft-skinned ambulances
are integral to this organization, as is staffing for a true aeromedical
capability. The only HSS capability shortfall remaining is that of a
dedicated aeromedical evacuation platform, and this is a requirement
common to all Roles of CF HSS that the CF must still address.

In the context of the CF Force Planning Scenarios, the evolved CF field ambulance, seamlessly augmentable on a task-tailored basis and highly mobile, is indeed well-situated to provide deployed HSS in scenarios from operations other than war to warfighting. It will, therefore, be a key capability for land casualty management in the patient care continuum across the spectrum of conflict in the 21st century battlespace.

ANNEX A – CF FORCE PLANNING SCENARIOS*

```
PEACE                          CONFLICT
┌─────────────────────────────────────────┐
│ OPERATIONS OTHER THAN WAR                │
└─────────────────────────────────────────┘
                                    ┌──────────────────┐
                                    │     WARFIGHTING  │
                                    └──────────────────┘
┌──────────────┐
│ SAR          │
└──────────────┘
┌──────────────┐
│ Disaster Relief │
└──────────────┘
┌────────────────────────────┐
│ Int'l Humanitarian Assistance │
└────────────────────────────┘
┌──────────────────────────────────────┐
│ Surv & Control of Cdn Territory & Approaches │
└──────────────────────────────────────┘
┌──────────────────────────────┐
│ Evacuation of Canadians Overseas │
└──────────────────────────────┘
┌──────────────────────────────┐
│ Peace Support Operations (Chapter 6) │
└──────────────────────────────┘
┌──────────────────────────┐
│ Aid of the Civil Power   │
└──────────────────────────┘
┌──────────────────────────────────┐
│ National Sovereignty/Interest Enforcement │
└──────────────────────────────────┘
                    ┌──────────────────────────────┐
                    │ Peace Support Operations (Chapter 7) │
                    └──────────────────────────────┘
                        ┌──────────────────────────────┐
                        │ Defence of Canadian - US Territory │
                        └──────────────────────────────┘
                            ┌──────────────────┐
                            │ Collective Defence │
                            └──────────────────┘
┌──────────────────────────────┐
│ NON-COMBAT OPERATIONS        │
└──────────────────────────────┘
                        ┌──────────────────────────┐
                        │     COMBAT OPERATIONS    │
                        └──────────────────────────┘
```

* From DND, VCDS *Force Planning Scenarios* on the DND Director of Defence Analysis DWAN website vcds.mil.ca/dgsp/dda/scen/into_e.asp, accessed 17 Sep 2002.

No.	Scenario	Summary
1	Search and Rescue in Canada	Sub-scenarios include rescue from a ship at sea, search and rescue of an overdue hunting party in the North, and the rescue of survivors from a major airliner downed in a remote area in the North.
2	Disaster Relief in Canada	Assist in the relief of human suffering and help authorities to re-establish the local infrastructure after a major earthquake on the west coast of Canada.
3	International Humanitarian Assistance	As part of a UN operation, assist with the delivery of relief supplies to refugees amassed in a central African nation.
4	Surveillance/Control of Canadian Territory and Approaches	Assist Other Government Departments and law enforcement agencies in identifying, tracking and, if required, intercepting platforms suspected of carrying contraband goods or illegal immigrants before or after entering Canadian territory.
5	Protection and Evacuation of Canadians Overseas	Assist DFAIT, as part of a combined force, in the protection and evacuation of Canadian nationals in a foreign nation threatened by imminent conflict.
6	Peace Support Operations (Chapter 6)	Participate as part of a UN peacekeeping force maintaining a cease-fire and assisting in the creation of a stable and secure environment where peace building can take place.
7	Aid of the Civil Power	Assist civil authorities in the establishment of law and order in an area where lawlessness has occurred as the result of disputes over the control of water rights in a time of severe drought.
8	National Sovereignty/ Interests Enforcement	Claiming extended jurisdiction under UNCLOS III, Canada has requested the cessation of seabed exploitation operations by a foreign nation. The CF will assist OGDs in the enforcement of Canadian claims.
9	Peace Support Operations (Chapter 7)	At the request of a foreign nation, as part of a UN coalition, the CF will participate in operations to restore pre-conflict boundaries and return control of an occupied area to the control of the rightful country.
10	Defence of Canada/US Territory	In cooperation with US forces, the CF will defend Canada/US territory against potential threats initiated by an emerging world power as a result of Canadian and American support for a foreign military operation.
11	Collective Defence	As part of a NATO force, the CF will attempt to deter and, if necessary, contain an attack on NATO territory and conduct restoration operations.

ANNEX B - LEVELS OF HEALTH SERVICES SUPPORT*

General. HSS shall be organized into levels of support corresponding to the command and control relationship at each level of organization. Each successive level becomes more sophisticated from front to rear (see following section for descriptions of Roles of Health Care).

Tactical Support at the Unit Level. Medical and/or dental elements attached or integral to units (normally Role 1 HSS, but may be augmented), e.g., ship's sickbay, unit medical station or squadron medical element.

Tactical Support at the Environment Component Level. HSS elements attached or integral to lower level environmental formations (normally Role 2 HSS, but may be augmented), e.g., fleet auxiliary logistic support ship, field ambulance or airfield medical station.

Operational Level Support. HSS elements operationally responsible to the Canadian Task Force (TF) Commander of CNC (through TF Support Group/ National Support Element [NSE] Commander) (normally Role 3 HSS, but may be augmented), e.g., Composite Health Services Unit.

Strategic Level Support. Normally, Canada-based health services formations and units, e.g., CFHSG, HSGs, maritime HS units, CFEME and CMED (normally Role 4 HSS), but may be augmented. In exceptional circumstances, strategic level support could be derived from allied military and foreign nation capabilities provided health care delivery meets Canadian levels of accessibility and quality of health care.

---

* DND, *Health Services Support to Canadian Forces Operations*, B-GG-005-004/AF-017, draft dated August 2002 (Ottawa: DND, 2002), paragraph 111.

ANNEX C - ROLES OF HEALTH CARE[*]

GENERAL

In addition to levels of support, HSS shall also be based on clinical capabilities designed to meet the characteristics of the operational environment and to play a specific part in force health protection and the progressive examination, treatment, evacuation and hospitalization of sick and injured personnel. These capabilities are referred to as "Roles" and are relative to medical and dental care. A capability may be enhanced to meet the specific requirements of a mission by the selection of selected capability modules, the presence of which is indicated by the "+" sign (e.g., Role 2+).

As a general rule, as HSS capabilities are increased, it is at the price of increased requirements for complex equipment, personnel and supplies, which in turn increases lift and other support. Highly sophisticated treatment facilities in combat areas could encumber the commander and restrict his freedom of movement. However, if the nature of the operation allows it, sophisticated treatment facilities can be positioned near to the most likely point(s) of injury/onset of illness.

The number and types of HSS treatment facilities and their location will be determined by the casualty and patient/workload estimates and the time required for transportation from point of injury/onset of illness to the required treatment capability, keeping in mind the time-related constraint of medical care. The availability and type of transport assets to be utilized, the length and difficulty of the evacuation route, the operational environment and its limitations, and the operational level evacuation policy will have an impact on the size and capabilities of treatment facilities.

ROLES OF MEDICAL CARE

ROLE 1. The minimum capabilities of this role include locating casualties, providing them with first aid and emergency medical care, evacuating them from the site of injury to a safer location, sorting them

---

[*]   DND, *Health Services Support to Canadian Forces Operations*, B-GG-005-004/AF-017, draft dated August 2002 (Ottawa: DND, 2002), paragraphs 112 and 901.

according to treatment precedence, and stabilizing and preparing them for evacuation to the next Role of care, if required.

ROLE 2. The minimum capabilities of this role emphasize efficient and rapid evacuation of stabilized patients from supported elements, and en route sustaining care. Emergency lifesaving resuscitative procedures may be performed. Patients requiring minor care may be held for short periods and returned to duty. Medical resupply may be provided to supported Role 1 facilities. Role 2 capabilities may be augmented to include capacities for emergency surgery, intensive care, essential post-operative care, blood replacement, diagnostic services, and stress reaction and mental health management.

ROLE 2+. This consists of the Role 2 minimum capability augmented by any or all of the following: life/limb-saving surgery, intensive care, essential postoperative care, blood replacement, laboratory services, basic diagnostic imaging capability.

ROLE 3. The minimum capabilities of this role emphasize resuscitation, initial wound surgery, post-operative care, and short-term surgical and medical in-patient care. Diagnostic services such as x-ray and laboratory, and limited-scope internal medicine and psychiatric services, are available. In-theatre reception and storage of medical supplies and blood, and distribution to supported units, is provided, as well as repair of medical equipment within the area of operations. Other ancillary capabilities include liaison teams for tracking Canadian patients in allied or host-nation facilities, teams providing assistance with stress reaction and mental health management, and coordination of force health protection activities in the area of operations. Role 3 capabilities may be augmented with specialist surgical (neurosurgical, maxillofacial surgical, burns etc.) capabilities, advanced and specialist diagnostic capabilities (CT scan, arthroscopy, sophisticated laboratory tests, etc.), major medical, dental and nursing specialties, and environmental health and industrial hygiene capabilities.

ROLE 4. This Role includes reconstructive surgery, definitive care hospitalization, rehabilitation, storage and distribution of national medical stocks inclusive of blood, blood products and intravenous fluids, and major repair or replacement of medical equipment.

ROLES OF DENTAL CARE

ROLE 1 (Emergency Care). This capability is the most basic type of dental care. It consists of services rendered to treat acute conditions (pain, infection and trauma), to control life-threatening oral circumstances (hemorrhage and respiratory distress) and to initially stabilize, for evacuation, injuries to the teeth, jaws and associated orofacial structures. Common examples of Role 1 dental care include extractions, placement of sedative/temporary restorations, therapeutic medication by injection or prescription, and application of pressure dressings.

ROLE 2 (Sustaining Care). This Role includes the treatments required to address emergency casualty situations, as well as therapies to deal with additional urgent oral conditions and those measures required to intercept potential dental casualties. This support aims to minimize time lost to personnel engaged in operations. Common examples of diagnoses which require Role 2 care include decayed teeth, defective restorations, tooth fractures, acute periodontal (gum) conditions, traumatic and inflammatory oral lesions, pericoronitis (infected wisdom teeth), temporomandibular joint (TMJ) disorders (acute or chronic non-surgical management), post-operative surgical complications and endodontic (root canal) conditions. Role 2 care includes diagnostic services (examinations, radiographs, laboratory tests), temporary and basic restorations, tooth extractions, pulpectomies (the initial stage of root canal therapy), routine denture adjustments (e.g., repairs or additions), debridement of oral lesions, gingival curettage, written referrals/consults and counseling as well as the initial stabilization of oral and maxillofacial fractures and injuries in preparation for evacuation.

ROLE 3 (Maintaining Care). Role 3 intervention seeks to maintain the overall fitness of personnel at functional fitness status (NATO Level 2). This allows for the operational deployment of personnel without the need of routine care. While Role 3 care includes the same types of procedures provided in Role 2 care, time and space permit more time-consuming and complex treatments and the active role of specialists where required. Role 3 care includes more definitive management of maxillofacial injuries, as well as restorative (fillings), oral surgical (extractions), periodontal (gum disease), endodontic (root canals), prosthodontic (dentures) and preventative (cleaning/oral health education) services.

ROLE 4 (Rehabilitative Care). Role 4 functions provide a full range of dental services, including comprehensive rehabilitative care. It aspires to repair and restore deficits in full oral function (including aesthetics) incurred because of wounds or disease. Examples of Role 4 care include complex endodontics, extensive restorative dentistry, prosthodontics (complex bridges and dentures, and osseointegrated implants), periodontal surgery, complex surgical procedures (jaw repair/realignment), complex TMJ therapy, speech-aid appliances, and maxillofacial prosthodontics.

NOTES

1   US Department of Defense (DoD), Medical Readiness Review Group, *Medical Readiness Planning in the US European Command*, US DoD Report 93-INS-13 (Washington:DoD, 1984), iii. When the report was published, Zimble was the US Navy's Senior Medical Inspector and a future US Navy Surgeon General.

2   Canada, Department of National Defence (DND), *Canadian Joint Task List* (version 1.4) (Ottawa: Directorate of Defence Analysis, 2001).

3   DND, VCDS *Force Planning Scenarios* on the DND Director of Defence Analysis DWAN website vcds.mil.ca/dgsp/dda/scen/into_e.asp, accessed 17 Sep 2002.

4   P.W. Lund, "Medical Support for Future Combat: No more Vietnams," *Naval War College Review* 45, no. 2 (Spring 1992), 80-92.

5   A.M. Smith and C.H. Llewellyn, "Tactical and Logistical Compromise in the Management of Combat Casualties: There is no Free Lunch!" *Naval War College Review* 43, no. 1 (Winter 1990), 53-66.

6   S.F. Gouge, *Combat Health Support of the Transformation Force in 2015*, (Carlisle Barracks, PA: US Army War College, 2001), 21.

7   US Army Medical Department (AMEDD), *AMEDD After Next Joint Medical Wargame 2000: Final Report* (San Antonio, TX: US AMEDD Centre & School, 2000), 2.

8   M.J.Conversino, "Sawdust Superpower: Perceptions of US Casualty Tolerance in the Post-Gulf War Era," *Strategic Review* 25, no. 1 (Winter 1997), 15-23.

9   DND, *Health Services Support to Canadian Forces Operations*, B-GG-005-004/AF-017, draft dated August 2002, (henceforth *HSS to CF Ops*) (Ottawa: DND, 2002), paragraph (para) 209.

10   DND, *HSS to CF Ops*, para 111; and North Atlantic Treaty Organization (NATO), *Allied Joint Medical Support Doctrine* (Ratification Draft 1), *AJP-4.10* (henceforth *AJP-4.10*) (Casteau, Belgium: Supreme Headquarters Allied Powers Europe, 1999), para 105.

11   NATO, *AJP-4.1*, para 113; and *HSS to CF Ops*, paras 112 and 901.

12   DND, Canadian Forces Health Services (CFHS), *Medical Support to the Army*, briefing note prepared by DHO 2-2 for COS HS dated 6 March 1997; and D.A. Salisbury, "Prescription 2020: Considerations for a Military Medical Strategy for the Canadian Forces," paper written for National Security Studies Course (NSSC) 4 (Toronto: Canadian Forces College, October 2002), 19-20.

13   NATO, *AJP-4.10*, para 115.

14   DND, *HSS to CF Ops*, para 110(1)(b).

15   DND, Director General Health Services, *Standing Committee on Operational Medicine Review: Phase One Final Report* (henceforth *SCOMR 1*) (Ottawa: CFHS, 2001), para 2.

16   NATO, *AJP-4.10*, para 107(2/3).

17   NATO, *AJP-4.10*, para 206(2).

18   University of Maryland, "R. Adams Cowley Shock Trauma Center," University of Maryland Medical System website www.ummscareers.com/r_adams_cowley.htm, accessed 14 September 2002.

19   E.B. Lerner and R.M. Moscati, "The Golden Hour: Scientific Fact or Medical 'Urban Legend'?" *Academic Emergency Medicine* 9, no. 7 (2002), 760; M. Schinco and J.J. Tepas, "Beyond the Golden Hour: Avoiding the Pitfalls from Resuscitation to Critical Care," *Surgical Clinics of North America* 82, no. 2 (April 2002), 325-32; and B.E. Bledsoe, "The Golden Hour: Fact or Fiction," *Emergency Medical Services* 31, no. 6 (June 2002),105.

20   J.M. Tallon, "The Golden Hour Paradigm," *Academic Emergency Medicine* 8, no. 7 (2001), 758-60; J.E. George snd M.S. Quattrone, "The Golden Hour: Trauma Center Standards in Non-trauma-Center Emergency Departments," *Journal of Emergency Nursing* 17, no. 5 (October 1991), 332; and S. Toulson, "A Guide to Advanced Trauma Life Support," *Professional Nurse* 9, no. 2 (November 1993), 95-7.

21   DND, *HSS to CF Ops*, paras 202(4), 203(2); and NATO, AJP-4.10, para 109(2).

22   American College of Surgeons Committee on Trauma, *ATLS Student Course Manual*, 6ᵗʰ ed. (Chicago: American College of Surgeons, 1997), 9-12.

23   D.D.Trunkey, "Trauma," *Scientific American* 249, no. 2 (1983), 20-7.

24   United Kingdom (UK), *Joint Medical Doctrine*, Joint Warfare Publication 4-03 (henceforth *UK JWP 4-03*) (Shrivenham: UK Joint Doctrine & Concepts Centre), para 306.

25   DND, *HSS to CF Ops*, pp. GL-6, GL-8.

26   A.M. Smith, "All Bleeding Stops Eventually," *US Naval Institute Proceedings* 127, no. 11 (November 2001), 68-71.

27   R.M. Hardaway, *Care of the Wounded in Vietnam* (Manhattan, KS: Sunflower University Press, 1988), 6.

28   D.C. Grossman, et al., "Urban-rural Differences in Pre-hospital Care of Major Trauma," *Journal of Trauma* 42, no. 4 (April 1997), 723-9.

29   DND, *HSS to CF Ops*, para 203; and NATO, *AJP-4.10*, para 109.

30   DND, *HSS to CF Ops*, para 109(1)(f).

31   A.M. Smith and C.H. Llewellyn, "Caring for our Casualties," *US Naval Institute Proceedings* 117, no. 12 (December 1991), 72-8.

32   M. Hammick, "The Cutting Edge: Battlefield Casualty Management," *International Defense Review* 25, no. 3 (1993), 243-51.

33   Smith and Llewellyn, "Caring for our Casualties," 72-8.

34   L.W. Grau snd W.A. Jorgensen, "Handling the Wounded in a Counter-guerrilla War: The Soviet/Russian Experience in Afghanistan and Chechnya," *US Army Medical Department Journal* (January-February 1998), 2-9.

35   NATO, *AJP-4.10*, paras 109, 111(2).

36   DND, *HSS to CF Ops*, para 209(6).

37   US Army, *Health Service Support in a Theater of Operations*, Field Manual 8-10 (henceforth *US Army FM 8-10*) (Washington: Department of the Army, 1991), paras 4-9, 5-9.

38   US Air Force, *Health Services*, Air Force Doctrine Document 2-4.2 (Maxwell AFB: US Air Force Doctrine Center, 1999), 9; and US Air Force Air Combat Command Office of the Command Surgeon website, *EMEDS System*, www.sg.langley.af.mil, accessed 30 Sep 2002.

39   US Navy, *Operational Health Service Support*, Naval Warfare Publication 4-02 (Norfolk: Naval Doctrine Command, 1995), para 1.5.2.

40   US Marine Corps, *Health Service Support Operations*, Marine Corps Warfighting Publication 4-11.1 (henceforth *USMC MCWP 4-11.1*) (Washington: US Department of the Navy, 1998), paras 3002, 8003.

41   J.H.B. Peay, III, "Correlating Medical Forces Forward," *Joint Forces Quarterly* 14 (Winter 1996-97), 70-4.

42   *SCOMR 1*, para 258, Annex P paras 30-31.

43   DND, *HSS to CF Ops*, paras 309(1), 906, 908(5).

44   Ibid., para 915(4)(d).

45   Lund, "Medical Support for Future Combat," 80-92.

46   NATO, *AJP-4.10*, para 113.

47   W.P. Thornton and J.C. Neubauer, "United Nations Aeromedical Evacuation Operations in the Former Yugoslavia," in *NATO Advisory Group for Aerospace Research & Development Proceedings 554*, AGARD publication AGARD-CP-554 (Neuilly-sur-Seine, France: NATO, 1995), pp. 3-1 to 3-7.

48   US AMEDD, *Military Medical History* from correspondence course MD0405 (San Antonio: US AMEDD Centre & School, 2002), paras 2-10, 2-16, 3-4.

49   R.L. DeHart, ed., *Fundamentals of Aerospace Medicine* (Philadelphia: Lea & Febiger, 1985), 601.

50   "The Beginnings of Military Transportation by Air, Part I: 1917-1929," *Journal of the American Aviation Historical Society* 44, no. 4 (Winter 1999), 242-54.

51   C.H. Briscoe, "Helicopters in Combat: World War II," *Special Warfare* 14, no. 3 (Summer) (2001), 32-8.

52   K. Finlayson, "Helicopters in Combat: Korea," *Special Warfare* 14, no. 3 (Summer)(2001), 39-41.

53   P. Dorland and J. Nanney, *Dust Off: Army Aeromedical Evacuation in Vietnam* (Washington: US Army Center of Military History, 1982,) 4.

54   DeHart, ed., *Fundamentals of Aerospace Medicine*, 600.

55   US Army, *Employment of the Medical Company (Air Ambulance)*, Field Manual 8-10-26 (henceforth *US Army FM 8-10-26*) (Washington: US Department of the Army, 1999), p. 1-4b.

56   N.C. Mann, et al., "Injury Mortality Following the Loss of Air Medical Support for Rural Interhospital Transport," *Academic Emergency Medicine* 9, no. 7 (July 2002), 694-8; S.H. Thomas, et al., "Helicopter Transport and Blunt Trauma Mortality: A Multicenter Trial," *Journal of Trauma* 52, no. 1 (January) (2002), 136-45; W.A. Kerr, et al., "Differences in Mortality Rates among Trauma Patients Transported by Helicopter and Ambulance in Maryland," *Prehospital Disaster Medicine* 14, no. 3 (July-September 1999),159-64; and L.M. Jacobs, et al., "Helicopter Air Medical Transport: Ten-year Outcomes for Trauma Patients in a New England Program," *Connecticut Medicine* 63, no. 11 (November 1999), 677-82.

57   C. E. Braithwaite, et al., "A Critical Analysis of On-scene Helicopter Transport on Survival in a Statewide Trauma System," *Journal of Trauma* 45, no. 1 (July 1998), 140-4; P. Cunningham, et al., "A Comparison of the Association of Helicopter and Ground Ambulance Transport with the Outcome of Injury in Trauma Patients Transported from the Scene," *Journal of Trauma* 43, no. 6 (December 1997), 940-6; and V.L. Chappell, et al., "Impact of Discontinuing a Hospital-based Air Ambulance Service on Trauma Patient Outcomes," *Journal of Trauma* 52, no. 3 (March 2002), 486-91.

58   DND, *HSS to CF Ops*, paras 515(3)(a), 518, 907(4), 916(2)(c).

59   *SCOMR 1*, para 215; Annex P para 37.

60   NATO, *AJP-4.10*, paras 307(1)(a), 316(1).

61   DND, *HSS to CF Ops*, para 110(1)(b).

62   *SCOMR 1*, Annex E paras 133-136.

63   DND, CFHS, *Standing Committee on Operational Medicine Review: Phase Two - Aeromedical Evacuation Working Group Report* (Draft) (henceforth *SCOMR 2 AEWG*) (Ottawa: DND, 2002), para 3-5.

64   R.T. Gerhardt, et al., "US Army MEDEVAC in the New Millennium: A Medical Perspective," *US Army Medical Department Journal* (July-September 2000), 36-43; and R.T. Gerhardt, et al., "US Army MEDEVAC in the New Millennium: A Medical Perspective," *Aviation Space and Environmental Medicine* 72, no. 7 (July 2001), 659-64.

65   *US Army FM 8-10-26*, p. 1-5.

66   F.V. Bauer, "The Future of Helicopter Aeromedical Evacuation," *Marine Corps Gazette* 77, no. 9 (September 1993), 49-51.

67   US DoD, *Medical Mobilization Planning and Execution*, DoD report 93-INS-13 (Washington: DoD, 1993), 149-50.

68   US General Accounting Office (GAO), *Operation Desert Storm: Full Army Capability Not Achieved*, publication GAO/NSAID-92-175 (Washington: GAO, 1992), 45-9.

69   R.T. Gerhardt, et al., "US Army MEDEVAC in the New Millennium," *US Army Medical Department Journal*, 36-43.

70   J.A. Powell, *Aeromedical Evacuation: How Will We Clear the Next Battlefield?* (Carlisle Barracks: US Army War College, 2002), 7.

71   *USMC MCWP 4-11.1*, paras 3002, 8003.

72   US Navy, *Operational Health Service Support*, Naval Warfare Publication 4-02, para 1.5.2.

73   A.M. Smith, "Care Delayed is Care Denied: Casualty Handling in Littoral Operations," *Naval War College Review* 52, no. 4 (Autumn 1999), 109-21.

74   DND, *HSS to CF Ops*, paras 914(4)(c), 915(4)(e).

75   *SCOMR 2 AEWG*, paras 22, 23.

76   *SCOMR 1*, para 178; Annex E paras 133-136 ; Annex G paras 115, 120; Annex O para 11.

77   *HSS to CF Ops*, para 518.

78   NATO Standardization Agreement (STANAG) 3204 – *Aeromedical Evacuation*, 6th ed. (Brussels: NATO Military Agency for Standardization, 1999), Annex B, para 5.

79   Colonel C.R. Shelley, personal communication 17 Sep 2002. Colonel Shelley recently commanded 408 Tactical Helicopter Squadron that conducted extensive operations in the Balkans.

80   DND,1 Canadian Air Division HQ, data from Weather Section, Camp Black Bear, Velika Kladusa, Bosnia-Herzegovina via e-mail from A3 Met 2, 1 Cdn Air Div HQ, 17 Sep 2002.

81   Thornton and Neubauer, "United Nations Aeromedical Evacuation Operations in the Former Yugoslavia," pp. 3-1 to 3-7.

82   E. Krekorian, "Medical Procedures for a Changing Battlefield," *Marine Corps Gazette* 82, no. 5 (May 1998), 67-8.

83   W.F. Davis, "Cancel the MEDEVAC, He's Dead!" *Marine Corps Gazette* 77, no. 9 (September 1993), 45-7.

84   Bauer, "The Future of Helicopter Aeromedical Evacuation," 49-51.

85   Smith, "Care Delayed is Care Denied,"109-21.

86   Vietnam Helicopter Pilots Association (VHPA), *Helicopter Losses During the Vietnam War*, VHPA website www.vhpa.org/heliloss.pdf, accessed 15 Sep 2002.

87   D. Wood and M. Hewish, "The Falklands Conflict, Part 1: The Air War," *International Defence Review* 15, no. 8 (1982), 977-80.

88   A. Richard, *Military Incompetence: Why the American Military Doesn't Win*, (New York: Hill & Wang, 1985), 180-1.

89   G.M. Mullen, "Choppers Grounded," *US Army Aviation Digest* (September 1988), 5-14.

90   Smith, "Care Delayed is Care Denied,"109-21.

91   Lund, "Medical Support for Future Combat," 80-92; Smith and Llewellyn, "Caring for our Casualties," 72-8; S. Neel, *Medical Support of the US Army in Vietnam*, 1965-1970 (Washington: US Department of the Army, 1973), 50, 65, 121; and A.M. Smith, "The Influence of Medicine on Strategy," *Naval War College Review* 41, no. 2 (Spring 1988), 22-36.

92   Smith, "The Influence of Medicine on Strategy," 22-36.

93   J. Kitfield, "Combat Medicine," *Government Executive* 23, no. 1 (January1991), 22-31.

94   B. Eiseman, "The Next War: A Prescription," *US Naval Institute Proceedings* 101, no. 1 (January 1975), 30-7.

95   J.D. Stewart, "Evacuating the Wounded: Why it will be so Difficult," *Military Logistics Forum* 3, no. 1 (January-February 1986), 33.

96   D. Bolton, "Armour/anti-armour: The Future," *RUSI Journal* (Spring 1986), 32; A.M. Smith, "Until the First Bloodied Body Goes By," *US Naval Institute Proceedings* 119, no. 10 (October 1993), 64-9; Davis, "Cancel the MEDEVAC, He's Dead!" 45-7; Powell, *Aeromedical Evacuation*, 7; Smith, "The Influence of Medicine on Strategy," 22-36 and Kitfield, "Combat Medicine," 22-31.

97   R.D. Doughty, "Images of the Future Battlefield," *Military Review* 68, no. 1 (January 1988), 13.

98   Smith, "Care Delayed is Care Denied,"109-21.

99   Tallon, "The Golden Hour Paradigm," 758-60.

100   Dorland and Nanney, *Dust Off*,122-3.

101   Smith, "The Influence of Medicine on Strategy," 22-36.

102   C.G. Batty, "Changes in the Care of the Battle Casualty: Lessons Learned from the Falklands Campaign," *Military Medicine* 164, no. 5 (May 1999), 336-40.

103   C.J. Hooton, "Medical Support for the FMF: Far in the Rear, Too Much Gear," *Marine Corps Gazette* 74, no. 4 (April1990), 51-3; and Smith and Llewellyn, "Tactical and Logistical Compromise in the Management of Combat Casualties," 53-66.

104   Davis, "Cancel the MEDEVAC, He's Dead!" 45-7; and Bauer, "The Future of Helicopter Aeromedical Evacuation," 49-51.

105   NATO, *AJP-4.10*, paras 301(4)115, 308(1)(h).

106   DND, *HSS to CF Ops*, para 506(2).

107   Hammick, "The Cutting Edge: Battlefield Casualty Management," 243-51.

108   M.R. Gordon "Chechen Saboteurs Torch Russian Field Hospital," *The New York Times* (7 Jan 2000), 9-10.

109   J.F. Antal, "A Glimpse of Wars to Come: The Battle for Grozny," *Army* 49, no. 6 (June1990), 29-40; and L.W. Grau and T.L.Thomas, "'Soft Log' and Concrete Canyons: Russian Urban Combat Logistics in Grozny," *Marine Corps Gazette* 83, no. 10 (October1999), 67-75.

110   Grau and Thomas, "'Soft Log' and Concrete Canyons," 67-75.

111   *SCOMR 1*, para 20.

112   NATO, *AJP-4.10*, para 306(2).

113   *SCOMR 1*, paras 176, 177, 213; Annex E paras 11, 14; Annex G paras 122-124; Annex O paras 9, 10 ; Annex P para 35.

114   DND, *HSS to CF Ops*, paras 501(3)(a), 514(2).

115   CF Medical Group Headquarters, email from G3 Ops-2, dated 7 Oct 2002.

116   DND, "Wheeled Light Armoured Vehicle Life Extension Project," Capital Project #00000058 (Chief of Land Staff).

117   DND, "Wheeled Light Armoured Vehicle Life Extension Project – Bison Conversion Fielding Plan," 30058-102 (DLR3-5), dated July 2002, para 12.

118   DND, *HSS to CF Ops*, para 907(2).

119   Jane's Information Group, *Jane's Military Vehicles and Logistics 2002/2003* (Alexandria, VA: Jane's Information Group Inc., 2002).

120   P. Liston, "Casualty Evacuation Underpins Battlefield Medical Support," *Jane's International Defence Review* 31, no. 5 (May1998), 53-8.

121   Smith, "All Bleeding Stops Eventually," 68-71.

122   DND, *HSS to CF Ops*, para 915(3).

123   A.M. Smith and R.F. Bellamy, "Conceptual Errors in Combat Casualty Care Training," *Navy Medicine* (July-August 1988), 16.

124   NATO, *AJP-4.10*, para 110(1).

125   DND, *HSS to CF Ops*, para 109(1)(c).

126   *US Army FM 8-10*, para 4-6.

127   *UK JWP 4-03*, para 457.

128   DND, *HSS to CF Ops*, para 507(2)(b).

129   *USMC MCWP 4-11.1*, para 8001.

130   C.G. Blood, et al., "Comparison of Casualty Presentation and Admission Rates during Various Combat Operations," *Military Medicine* 159, no. 6 (June1994), 457-61.

131   Smith and Llewellyn, "Caring for our Casualties," 72-8.

132   R.T. Gerhardt, et al., "US Army MEDEVAC in the New Millennium," *US Army Medical Department Journal*, 36-43.

133   DoD, *Joint Tactics, Techniques and Procedures for Patient Movement in Joint Operations*, US Joint Publication 4-02.2 (Washington: US Joint Staff, 1996); NATO, *AJP-4.10*, para 115; *UK JWP 4-03*, para 457; and DND, *HSS to CF Ops*, para 315(2).

134   *UK JWP 4-03*, para 457.

135   Powell, *Aeromedical Evacuation*, 7.

136   DND, *HSS to CF Ops*, para 521.

137   NATO, *AJP-4.10*, para 301(4).

138   Mullen, "Choppers Grounded,"5-14.

139   DND, *HSS to CF Ops*, paras 510(3), 516(1).

140   DND, *HSS to CF Ops*, para 209(6).

141   Liston, "Casualty Evacuation Underpins Battlefield Medical Support,"53-8.

CHAPTER 4

BLURRING OF THE LINES:
THE CALL FOR AN INTEGRAL SURGICAL CAPABILITY
IN CANADIAN FIELD AMBULANCES

Lieutenant-Colonel David R. Weger

INTRODUCTION

As visions of the future battlespace dance in the heads of academic and military thinkers alike, a clearer picture of what that battlespace will look like and of what our forces will have to look like to operate effectively in it is beginning to emerge. While the full picture remains murky, what we know for certain is that future military operations will continue to generate combat casualties who will have to be rescued from their place of injury, quickly stabilized, and rapidly evacuated to an appropriate level of care. What will change, and indeed is already beginning to change, is our understanding of how quickly and aggressively we will have to deliver care in order to assure the survival of these casualties. This will demand lightweight, very mobile Health Service Support (HSS) elements that can operate as close to the fighting as the tactical situation allows and provide resuscitative surgery to stabilize casualties for further evacuation.

Canadian operational HSS doctrine in respect of Far Forward Surgery no longer supports our emerging picture of military operations in the future battlespace. Therefore, it will be argued here that it is time to redefine the way in which we have grouped operational care capabilities, to include initial resuscitative surgery as a Role 2 function. It will then be argued that a Far Forward Surgery capability as an integral element of our existing brigade group field ambulances should be established as part of this redefinition. The chapter will first establish a general context for the discussion, present a view of HSS in tomorrow's battlespace, describe the structure of operational HSS and briefly discuss the physiologic nature of trauma as defined by the "Golden Hour." It will then go on to analyze the evacuation of casualties from the battlefield, examine the historical employment of Far Forward Surgery, and assess the failings of our current doctrine and organizational structures with respect to Far Forward Surgery. The chapter will conclude by presenting a model for the way ahead in Far Forward Surgery, detailing the advantages inherent in the proposed model and identifying three supporting imperatives upon which the success of a true Far Forward Surgery capability is predicated.

CONTEXT AND DEFINITIONS

While this chapter directly addresses one aspect of sustainment to tactical level land operations, the topic itself transcends merely tactical consider-ations. It does so in that a viable operational HSS capability provides our soldiers with the assurance that should they be injured in combat they will receive quick and appropriate medical attention. This assurance has a powerful effect on morale and as such, contributes to the cohesion sought by all operational-level commanders. Indeed, the link between viable HSS, morale and operational effectiveness was one upon which Field-Marshal Viscount Slim placed great emphasis during his command of the Allied forces in Burma during the Second World War.[1] The impor-tance of this link is echoed today in current North Atlantic Treaty Organization (NATO) joint doctrine, which cites HSS as a major contrib-utor to both morale and force protection.[2]

Although the subject of Far Forward Surgery enjoys a relatively compre-hensive treatment within international professional and technical literature, Canadian perspectives on the issue are quite sparse. Indeed, when the paper on which this chapter is based was written in October 2003, Salisbury and English's "Prognosis 2020: A Military Medical Strategy for the Canadian Forces" and Taylor's "Whither the Field Ambulance? Role 2 Land Health Service Support in the 21st Century Battlespace" appeared to be the only two recent examinations of the major issues facing HSS in the future battlespace.[3] As the title of Salisbury and English's paper implies, their treatment of the subject focuses on those factors that need to be considered in developing a longer-term strategy for HSS. In so doing, they highlight the importance of Far Forward Surgery, but envisage a future where near complete reliance on Forward Aeromedical Evacuation (defined in NATO doctrine as evacuation conducted by air between points within the combat zone[4]) renders today's field ambulances irrelevant.[5]

Taylor also stresses the importance of Far Forward Surgery, but contrary to Salisbury and English, he argues in favour of the continued relevance of the field ambulance as both an operating base for the attachment of Far Forward Surgery capabilities and for its continued capability of ground based casualty evacuation. Indeed, although Taylor clearly asserts that the establishment of a dedicated Canadian Forward Aeromedical Evacuation capability is essential to ensure effective HSS for the CF in the future battlespace, he contends that ground based evacuation will be also a required capability for casualty movement for the foreseeable future.[6]

Before proceeding with this discussion, the following definitions of Far Forward Surgery and resuscitative surgery will be applied here:

> **Far Forward Surgery** – resuscitative surgery conducted at, or forward of, a Role 2 HSS facility or unit (i.e., field ambulance level or forward).

> **Resuscitative Surgery** – emergency surgical interventions for exsanguinating hemorrhage, airway compromise, life threatening chest injuries, and some soft tissue and orthopedic injuries. It focuses on providing only those procedures necessary to preserve life and limb until more definitive surgical care can be delivered.[7]

HSS IN TOMORROW'S BATTLESPACE

Tomorrow's battlespace has been described as a place where technology offers increased lethality, which in turn will demand a high degree of mobility and great dispersion of increasingly decentralized operational elements.[8] Speed, agility and flexibility will be the keys to survival in an environment where smaller but more capable groups of soldiers come together to accomplish specific missions and then quickly disperse again for protection.[9] The distinction between front and rear, close and deep, will blur as the increased range and accuracy of long-range weapons forces large installations operating in divisional and corps rear areas to move further from the fight or risk annihilation.[10]

The battlespace envisioned above will have a significant impact on the delivery of operational HSS. As combat elements grow smaller and more dispersed, the reduced population at risk will result in fewer casualties and decrease the overall requirement for in-theatre "bed spaces." This trend will be supported by the increased speed with which combat forces are deployed into and out of operational theatres, thereby reducing the period of exposure to environmental and other factors that cause non-battle injuries. Concurrently, however, dispersion will increase evacuation distances, a factor that will be further exaggerated as larger surgical facilities move rearward to assure their survival.[11] These factors together will demand that resuscitative surgery be provided routinely far forward in order to stabilize casualties prior to lengthy evacuation, a requirement reinforced by Grau and Gbur:

> If sophisticated care could be quickly delivered near the scene of the injury, the need for early evacuation and all of the accompanying problems may be significantly reduced.[12]

In the future, forward deployed HSS elements will have to be lighter and highly mobile in order to keep pace with combat forces as they move within the fluid battlespace.[13] Agility and flexibility will become particularly critical in asymmetric environments, as HSS elements will need to swiftly concentrate assets as casualty densities develop during battle.[14] Such flexibility and responsiveness will only be achievable through the decentralization of resources and the enhancement of care capabilities at lower levels in the chain of casualty care. In tomorrow's dispersed operating environment, we will not be able to afford the economies of scale traditionally achieved by larger medical units.[15]

Beaty believes that ultimately it will be technology that allows "brilliant medics" to deliver highly sophisticated care very near the point of injury, thereby reducing the complications that arise as a consequence of delayed evacuation. The technology and techniques available to these "brilliant medics" will allow them to provide lifesaving interventions that today can only be provided on the operating table. That said, even the availability of resuscitative surgery at the very point of injury will not get a casualty out of the battlespace without a robust and capable evacuation system to back it up. Further, while many of the technologies needed for the realization of Beaty's future are already in development, their availability for use in the battlespace remains distant.[16] In the interim, we will continue to be reliant on systems that require significant support structures. Consequently, we must reconsider our operational HSS doctrine to rationalize the way in which we will deliver care for the near future.

THE STRUCTURE OF OPERATIONAL HSS

Continuity in the care and treatment of personnel injured in combat is optimally achieved through a progressive, phased HSS system. Within the Canadian Forces (CF), this system extends from the point of injury in the combat zone, through successively more clinically capable levels of care, eventually terminating in Canada. Each level of care provides not only an incremental increase in capabilities, but is also wholly inclusive of the capabilities of the level of care below it. Casualties move rearward through this system only so far as required to reach a level at which appropriate care can be provided to definitively deal with their medical condition. The capabilities resident at each level of the system are referred to as "Roles" and are classified by minimum capability requirements. The Roles are described in detail in Annex C to Chapter 3 in this volume.

The phased approach to casualty management presented above can be traced back to the Napoleonic and American Civil War periods, as described in Chapter 3. While the number of levels and specific capabilities included in each nation's or service's approach may vary, the general model remains in use within most major militaries. Although levels of care can be bypassed to move a patient directly to the required level of care, this is not routinely done. Indeed, senior American commanders, including the former Commander-in-Chief of US Central Command General Binford Peay III, have specifically cited the continued relevance of a phased care system on the modern battlefield.[17]

THE GOLDEN HOUR

The term "Golden Hour" is used within medical circles in reference to that period of time following injury within which a significant number of serious trauma casualties will die without surgical intervention. This model is based on civilian trauma data, which displays three peaks in a plot of deaths over time after injury: the first in the minutes immediately following injury, the second at one hour following injury and the third at six hours following injury (see Figure 3-1 in Chapter 3). Although some debate on the subject continues,[18] the one-hour window has come to be recognized as the civilian standard within which surgical intervention must be initiated to ensure the highest possible survival rates. The "Golden Hour" is also recognized as an appropriate benchmark within most military circles, including the CF, which states the following in its emerging joint HSS doctrine:

> Initial surgery, carried out as soon as possible after injury/onset of illness, ideally within the first hour, is the most important factor in reducing mortality rates and is the focal point of operational HSS.[19]

However, the doctrine manual goes on to note that it is unlikely that such a benchmark could be consistently achieved on operations,[20] a conclusion that is understandable given our current operational HSS structures.

The foregoing aside, there is also some debate as to the applicability of the "Golden Hour" within the realm of combat trauma. Indeed, examination of combat casualty data seems to point to the occurrence of the first peak of deaths as being at the 30 minute point, rather than at the one-hour point evident in the civilian trauma data.[21]

Smith goes so far as to suggest that as many as 20 percent of past combat fatalities suffered from injuries that were surgically correctable and might have lived had surgery been initiated within 30 minutes of injury.[22] Whether 30 minutes or 1 hour, it is clear that combat casualties must be promptly secured from the battlefield and rapidly evacuated to surgical care.

EVACUATION OF CASUALTIES

It has been generally accepted since the Vietnam War that the use of aviation assets is the most effective means of evacuating casualties from the battlefield. Indeed, it was during the Vietnam War that the ready availability of helicopters allowed development of the hub-and-spoke concept of evacuation. This concept, depicted in Figure 3-3 in Chapter 3, is highly dependent upon aviation assets to move casualties from any point in the evacuation chain directly to a Role 3 surgical care facility in the rear.

Taylor ably summarizes the potential perils of over reliance on such an aviation-centric model:

> While this approach has enjoyed successes in certain conflicts including the Vietnam War, and many periods during the last decade of peace support operations, history and doctrine recognize that it requires a tactically permissive environment, and may not be sufficiently resilient.[23]

Taylor's point on the vulnerability of aviation assets is a key one and well supported by historical precedent. During the Falklands Campaign the loss of helicopters, including several that were on evacuation missions, was a significant factor in the decision to deploy surgical assets ashore.[24] In the 1991 Persian Gulf War, US Marines found that heavy reliance on air evacuation was often hazardous[25] and during the Grenada Expedition the Americans lost in excess of 10 percent of their aviation assets. Even in Vietnam, where the Americans enjoyed air superiority and Forward Aeromedical Evacuation was very successfully employed, US forces lost a staggering 17,700 helicopters.[26] Lastly, the experiences of both the Russian forces in Grozny[27] and US forces in Mogadishu[28] revealed the fatal vulnerability and tenuous nature of helicopter evacuation in urban environments.

Nor is vulnerability to enemy action the only factor working against assured evacuation by air. The employment of aviation assets for evacuation missions can also be limited by weather, terrain, distance, availability and the medical condition of the casualty.[29] Hoff notes that, even when they are available, it often takes more than 30 minutes to get air evacuation assets to a casualty's location, which means that half of the time available to get the casualty to surgical care has already been consumed.[30]

The foregoing should not be construed as a blanket condemnation of Forward Aeromedical Evacuation in favour of ground based alternatives. Indeed, ground evacuation is also fraught with limitations that impact its ability to move casualties rapidly. Ground ambulances are inherently slower, limited by terrain, and particularly vulnerable to enemy attack in asymmetric environments and non-linear battlespaces. In the final analysis, the availability of dedicated air and ground evacuation assets is critical to casualty care, but both are vulnerable to disruption in today's likely operational environments. Furthermore, this reality is recognized within the Canadian Army as one that must be addressed as we move towards the *Interim Army*.[31]

FAR FORWARD SURGERY

The nature of the modern battlespace is such that it might well preclude the rapid evacuation of casualties to surgical facilities in rear areas. Yet the failure to adequately support casualties with initial stabilizing surgery within short timeframes causes premature death and long-term complications among those who do survive.[32] This leads one inexorably to the same conclusion drawn by Handy, Hooton, Lund and others - that we need to place surgically capable elements closer to the fight.[33] However, the ability of forward surgical elements to remain close to forward forces in a fluid battlespace demands that these elements be light, mobile and focused on providing only that minimal surgery required to ensure that the casualty makes it to the next destination in the chain of evacuation.[34]

The idea of pushing surgical assets forward to compensate for extended or delayed evacuation of casualties is not a new one. In both the Pacific and European Theatres during the Second World War, amphibious land-ing ships were converted for use as surgical suites and beached to provide forward stabilizing surgery before casualties were evacuated to care afloat.[35]   Forward surgical teams were also widely employed in Burma to compensate for the prolonged evacuation times associated with jungle operations.[36] During the Falklands Campaign, the vulnerability of afloat surgical assets and uncertainty of air evacuation prompted the British to deploy ad hoc surgical teams ashore. Indeed, as the campaign developed, surgical teams were extensively employed at the field ambulance level so as to more closely support combat operations.[37] Soviet forces in Afghanistan enjoyed a marked improvement in casualty survival rates once surgical capabilities were placed as far forward as possible, often down to the regimental level.[38]

Although the Persian Gulf War of 1991 revealed several major problem areas in US HSS doctrine and equipment, it also proved the utility of Far Forward Surgery on the modern battlefield. This was confirmed during

US military operations in Panama, for which the only in-theatre surgical capability was resident in the surgical elements attached to Echelon II units (the US equivalent of Canadian Role 2). The Panama conflict is also noteworthy because of the rapid evacuation of post-surgical patients out of theatre, whereas the long held belief had been that such patients required a significant period of immobility prior to extended evacuation.[39] Most recently, US forces deployed on both Operation Enduring Freedom in Afghanistan and Operation Iraqi Freedom employed Far Forward Surgery extensively, often down to battalion level.[40] In summary then, the requirement for and successful use of Far Forward Surgery enjoys substantial historical precedent.

EXISTING DOCTRINE

Despite the proven efficacy of Far Forward Surgery and its routine employment at Role 2 equivalent levels and below, there is a perplexing institutional reluctance to ascribe an organic surgical capability so far down the HSS chain. Indeed, current Canadian Army doctrine acknowledges that initial surgery should be performed as far forward as possible, but specifically recognizes this care capability as being inherently a Role 3 function.[41] Although the doctrine does note in passing the possible attachment of Forward Surgical Teams to Role 2 elements for the provision of initial surgery, it appears to exclude such an option by describing initial surgery as:

> ...that which must be performed urgently and as far forward as the tactical situation permits, with resuscitative and stabilizing surgical intervention in order to save life and limb, and to control hemorrhage and infection. It demands comprehensive pre-operative diagnostic procedures, intensive preparation for surgery, ... properly equipped operating room, appropriate post-operative care, and is characteristic of Role 3 treatment facilities.[42]

The treatment of Far Forward Surgery does not fare much better in emerging Canadian joint HSS doctrine, wherein the possible augmentations to the Role 2 capability are significantly increased, but remain additions rather than integral capabilities.[43] The logic of this approach would appear to be drawn from the Standing Committee on Operational

Medicine Support, which recommended that operationally deployed CF Task Forces be supported by a combined Role 1 and 2 HSS unit augmented with a surgical capability.[44] Indeed, it is exactly this type of arrangement that has been applied on most of the riskier land operations in which Canada has participated over the past decade, including the early Bosnia missions, Somalia, and now Afghanistan. In all three of these instances, the surgical capability attached to the integral Role 1 and 2 HSS elements was based on a reduced Advance Surgical Centre from 1 Canadian Field Hospital – a Role 3 unit.

Despite the fact that the US recognizes in doctrine and practice that initial resuscitative surgery is an Echelon II capability,[45] the US Army has done only marginally better than the CF in establishing such a capability as an integral Echelon II component. Indeed, US Army doctrine largely deals with the issue in much the same way as CF doctrine, with the attachment of Forward Surgical Teams from Echelon III to Echelon II units.[46] However, the US Army has long recognized the need for an integral Echelon II surgical capability for their Independent Brigade Combat Teams (IBCTs), the structure and operational capabilities of which resemble those resident in Canadian Mechanized Brigade Groups.[47] Furthermore, the surgical capabilities integral to the Brigade Support Medical Companies supporting US IBCTs are significantly more robust than those in the Forward Surgical Teams, a factor that has led to some criticism of the latter.[48]

The US Marine Corps has been much more progressive in its doctrinal dealings with Far Forward Surgery, in that it defines resuscitative surgery as an Echelon II capability and has established this capability as an integral component of all its medical battalions.[49] That said, as part of its doctrinal revisions in the mid-1990s as part of the Operational Maneuver from the Sea (OMFTS) concept, the Marine Corps seriously considered eliminating its shore-based surgical capabilities. This suggestion generated significant debate and strong cautions that doing so would likely make OMFTS unsupportable from an HSS perspective.[50] It is also worth considering that, although integral Echelon II surgical capabilities survived OMFTS doctrinal revisions, they may not fare so well as the Marine Corps tackles how it will support its latest doctrinal concept – Ship-to-Objective Maneuver.

NATO joint doctrine clearly recognizes the importance of timeliness in the provision of emergency care and notes that "[w]here emergency surgery can be provided forward the number of casualties saved can be increased, and the degree of disability can be minimized."[51] Despite this recognition, NATO doctrine goes on to classify such emergency surgery as a Role 3 capability that can be pushed forward to augment Role 2 units as required.[52] Indeed, NATO doctrine on the matter is so similar to CF joint doctrine that it is clear the former has served as a major guide in the development of the latter.

ASSESSING THE STATUS QUO

Before delving into any discussion on the way ahead for the employment of Far Forward Surgery in the CF, it is prudent to examine in what ways our current doctrine and organization fail to meet the requirements of the emerging battlespace. Consistent with CF doctrine, Canada's field surgical assets are currently resident in 1 Canadian Field Hospital, a 116-bed "cadre" unit based in Petawawa. This unit is composed of an 86-bed main facility, two 15-bed Advance Surgical Centres (ASCs), an Evacuation Company of two Ambulance Platoons and an Air Staging Facility, and a Forward Medical Equipment Depot. 1 Canadian Field Hospital is in the final years of a multi-year project to create a credible CF Role 3 operational HSS capability and as such is well equipped with modern technologies. However, the complexity of these technologies demands a high price in supporting personnel, equipment and supplies, which in turn significantly reduce the unit's agility. 1 Canadian Field Hospital is also a particularly heavy field unit and, although moveable, is not mobile given that it does not possess sufficient integral transport to move all of its assets in a single lift. From the surgical perspective, the purpose of the unit is to prepare patients for evacuation out of theatre by stabilizing them sufficiently to survive the rigors of extended flight. The level of surgical care and associated support systems required to do so are therefore more advanced than those required to provide forward resuscitative surgery.[53]

From the above description of 1 Canadian Field Hospital, it can be readily discerned that the unit's main facility is not capable of the mobility required to remain in contact with supported troops in a fluid environment. Indeed, such a conclusion is supported by an examination

of the performance of US Army Combat Surgical Hospitals, which closely approximates the structure and capabilities of 1 Canadian Field
Hospital but on a larger scale, during the 1991 Persian Gulf War.[54]
Furthermore, given its size and lack of mobility, it can also be concluded
that 1 Canadian Field Hospital is not capable of operating far enough
forward to provide a timely resuscitative surgery capability without
compromising its survival. This is recognized in our current Army
doctrine which notes the requirement for field hospitals to be far enough
to the rear so as to be out of enemy artillery range,[55] while our emerging
joint doctrine identifies its placement on the battlefield as being between
30 and 100 kilometers from the Forward Edge of the Battle Area.[56]

If 1 Canadian Field Hospital's main facility is incapable of providing the
Far Forward Surgery capabilities required in the emerging battlespace,
what of its ASCs? These sub-units are comprised of 109 personnel and
29 vehicles. They take approximately six hours to set up or tear down and
are described in doctrine as compact versions of the main facility. ASCs
are fully mobile with integral lift and are capable of operating independently for periods of up to 72 hours, in either a step-up capacity for the
main facility or to provide a surgical capability further forward than
would otherwise be prudent with the main facility. In this latter capacity
they are intended to provide Close Support to tactical formations.[57]

Although the above description of the CF's ASCs would appear to better
incorporate the characteristics necessary for a viable Far Forward Surgery
element, these sub-units would fare only marginally better in meeting our
needs than does 1 Canadian Field Hospital's main facility. The ASC's size
and mobility make it more suited to operating in forward areas than the
Field Hospital, but the six-hour set up time would inhibit its ability to
maintain proximity with supported forces in a fluid environment. Even
at its existing size, the ASC is still too heavy to either assure its survival
as far forward as it would have to operate to provide viable Far Forward
Surgery or to remain flexible enough to react quickly to changing operational situations. Indeed, the capabilities resident in the ASC are available
in much smaller configurations, including the Royal Netherlands Army
MOGOS (a Dutch acronym for mobile medical operating theatre system)
- a field surgical unit that is fully mobile on 13 vehicles and capable of
being operational within two hours at a distance of 10-15 kilometers from
the front line.[58] Even more impressive, and particularly well suited as a

potential integral Role 2 surgical capability, is the Advanced Surgical Suite for Trauma Casualties (ASSTC) fielded by the US Army and the US Marine Corps. This "hospital-in-a-box" with tent expansion offers triage, resuscitative surgery, post-operative care and temporary holding capabilities in a highly mobile package that can be operational within 15-30 minutes.[59]

THE WAY AHEAD FOR FAR FORWARD SURGERY

Overcoming our current shortfall in providing credible HSS on tomorrow's battlefield lies in part in improving the skill sets available to our first responders – the soldiers at section and platoon level. We need to place advanced lifesaving skills into the hands of those soldiers that will be first on the scene of combat injuries, because they are directly involved in the activities that generate them. Already well established within the US Army as the Combat Lifesaver program, this concept has proven its efficacy in operations[60] and been identified as a significant component in the provision of combat health support to the *US Army After Next*.[61] While such Tactical Combat Casualty Care (TCCC) trained soldiers remain first and foremost combat soldiers, they also provide a critical link between self/buddy aid and the Medical Technicians at company level. The need for such an enhancement to CF operational HSS capabilities has been recognized, endorsed by the Surgeon General and validated through a trial TCCC course conducted by 1 Canadian Mechanized Brigade Group during the spring of 2003.

Another key part of the overall solution lies in the development of our evacuation capabilities. A significant step in this direction is already well underway in the form of an ongoing project to reconfigure 77 Bison Wheeled Light Armored Vehicles as ambulances.[62] The attendant protection and mobility that this project brings to ground evacuation will significantly improve our ability to move casualties within tactical areas and maintain proximity to supported forces. Equally significant steps now need to be taken to secure dedicated Forward Aeromedical Evacuation assets, the lack of which limit our current and potential operational HSS capabilities.[63] Indeed, recent US operations in Iraq clearly link the success of Far Forward Surgery concepts to a robust and dedicated intra-theatre air evacuation capability.[64]

While implementing the foregoing requirements will further our ability to provide efficacious HSS in tomorrow's battlespace, the most critical task lies in creating a viable Far Forward Surgery concept. Such a concept must balance emerging demands for mobility, flexibility, capability and readiness. It must also be consistent with the direction in which the CF is moving at the operational and strategic levels. One solution that meets all of these requirements is the establishment of an integral resuscitative surgical capability within our existing field ambulances. The field element created to provide such a capability will by necessity have to be smaller than our current ASCs, but can inherently be smaller by virtue of being able to draw much of its first line support from existing field ambulance resources rather than having its own integral support assets. It will also have to be focused on providing only the resuscitative surgery necessary to ensure that casualties survive to the next destination in the chain of evacuation.

ADVANTAGES OF THE PROPOSED MODEL

The establishment of a surgical capability within Canadian field ambulances has a number of inherent advantages over current CF doctrinal and organizational practice. Foremost among these is that it will best meet the demands of tomorrow's battlefield by melding Far Forward Surgery capabilities into the existing framework of an operational element specifically tailored for the forward tactical environment. Ancillary advantages to be gained by implementation of the proposed model include improved cohesion, morale, training and readiness. As will be seen, a number of these advantages accrue as a result of having a formed, standing operational entity rather than generating deployable surgical capabilities on a case-by-case basis as is currently done in the CF.

Improved Mobility and Capability. Given its nature as a tactical field force unit, the field ambulance possesses an inherent mobility, which coupled with the depth resident in its multiple platoons, provides a flexibility to react quickly to changing operational conditions. The establishment of a surgical capability within such a unit provides an opportunity to capitalize upon these characteristics. That said, there is an inherent dichotomy between capability and mobility, and the very assets needed to sustain a Far Forward Surgery capability can significantly limit a unit's ability to keep pace with the very forces it is supporting. As such, we cannot simply transplant our existing ASCs from 1 Canadian Field Hospital to the field ambulances and must instead develop a lighter less logistically dependent Far Forward Surgery element. Thus, while the marriage of a surgical capability to the field ambulance presents a key opportunity, we must remain cognizant of Porr's caution that the highest priority remains mobility.[65]

Improved Command and Control. After Action Reports from US units in Afghanistan note the inherent difficulties that arise when external surgical elements are attached in support for the provision of Far Forward Surgery, particularly in respect of their unfamiliarity with the operating procedures of the units they are supporting.[66] Familiarity with procedures can only be achieved if supporting elements train with supported ones on an ongoing basis. The creation of an integral Far Forward Surgery capability in field ambulances would not only facilitate this, but would also ensure that the entire brigade-level HSS team remains focused on the needs of their affiliated brigade. It would also provide a capability to mount the full tactical-level HSS requirement for most contingency operations from a single unit, thereby streamlining the coordination of pre-and post-deployment activities. Furthermore, the integration of HSS assets is a significant factor in ensuring accomplishment of the HSS mission,[67] and although formalized command and control relationships facilitate such integration, it is best achieved when all HSS elements operating at the same level are unified under a single commander.

Improved Cohesion and Morale. Although a complete ASC has yet to be deployed operationally, Canada has deployed a surgical capability based on an ASC in support of several different operations over the past decade. Given the cadre structure of 1 Canadian Field Hospital, this has meant bringing together the constituent members of the unit at some point in advance of embarkation. However, the development of a team identity and the definition of individual roles within the team take time. This phenomenon is well recognized within military circles, wherein we invest a great deal of energy developing teamwork and group identity at all levels of our organization. The return on this investment is a highly cohesive team with strong morale, which is an important precursor to operational effectiveness. These outcomes are not achieved to the same degree when individuals are brought together on short notice prior to deployment and invariably their collective performance will be sub-optimal.[68] Further, cohesion is one of the main factors that have a consistent impact on reducing operational stress, a critical concern that must be duly considered by any organization with limited numbers of operational personnel.[69]

Improved Training. Under the current cadre structure of 1 Canadian Field Hospital, the HSS personnel that will staff surgical capabilities upon deployment do not have an opportunity to work regularly with the equipment they will use in the field. The lack of familiarity with equipment that results from this structure is regularly cited as a major operational issue, and has been specifically noted in US Army After Action Reports for the 1991 Persian Gulf War,[70] Kosovo[71] and most recently Afghanistan.[72] Collocating surgical personnel and equipment at the field ambulance level, thereby providing these personnel with the opportunity to work with field equipment on a regular basis, would largely overcome this issue. Nor would such an arrangement compromise wider specialist skill maintenance, as current CF practice in this area provides for time outside of purely clinical settings for the development of general military and operational skills.

Improved Readiness. Although the CF theoretically maintains an Immediate Reaction Force ASC, this facility is twice the size of a regular ASC and hence would be even less well suited than the latter for the provision of Far Forward Surgery support. Furthermore, the requirement to pull together the personnel to staff such a facility on short notice presents tremendous challenges, and invariably results in the late identification of personnel deficiencies. Consequently, the lack of a true standing Far Forward Surgery element limits our ability to react quickly to crises as they arise. The establishment of an integral Far Forward Surgical element at the field ambulance level would largely resolve this issue and allow for the rotation of some Immediate Reaction Force responsibilities among three units instead of one. It should also be noted that the advantages detailed above in respect of improved command and control, cohesion, morale and training, contribute directly to enhanced operational readiness.

Consistent with Future CF and Army Direction. Not surprisingly, a review of key strategic documents, like *Shaping the Future of the Canadian*

Forces: A Strategy for 2020[73] and *Advancing With Purpose: The Army Strategy*,[74] reveals some interesting themes relevant to this discussion. Replete with words like agile, capable, deployable and sustainable, these documents paint a future wherein the CF stands ready to deploy a relevant medium-weight force, in or out of a coalition, wherever deemed appropriate by the national authority. It is not too difficult to conclude from the foregoing that what is envisaged are globally deployable, early entry, self-sufficient brigade-size packages that must be ready to fight on arrival in-theatre. We have long realized that such brigade groups must be organically sustainable to be relevant, and the time has come to reappraise how self-sufficiency will be achieved on tomorrow's battlefield. As we have seen elsewhere in this chapter, self-sufficiency from the HSS perspective includes the ability to deploy a true Far Forward Surgery capability. This is best achieved, and our forces would be best supported, by establishing such a capability as an integral element of our brigade group field ambulances.

SUPPORTING IMPERATIVES

For an integral Role 2 Far Forward Surgery capability, as proposed here, to be successful, there are three major barriers that must be recognized and overcome. Doing so will not be easy, as all three of the associated supporting imperatives speak to issues that can be more widely classified as cultural, and cultural barriers are notoriously difficult overcome. First, although Canadian doctrine recognizes the requirement for hard choices to be made in treatment decisions within an operational environment,[75] our military physicians are products of a civilian medical system, which teaches them that compromise in patient care is never acceptable. Regrettably such compromises are an inherent reality in the provision of HSS during military operations and are critical to ensuring that the surgical assets we place far forward remain available to support those who can most benefit from them. In short, as noted by Smith:

> Surgeons in an echeloned system must accept the reality that they can render only the amount of care necessary for the moment, in stages, without attempting to carry out definitive care.[76]

Second, there is an existing paradigm within the Canadian military HS community that field hospitals must be state of the art and as comparable as possible to the capabilities of home-based fixed facilities. Such a belief inherently detracts from the imperative of providing appropriate HSS as early as possible (i.e., far forward) and focuses instead on building field-based medical centres.[77] Indeed, Porr stresses that combat surgery need not be as aseptic or as technologically advanced as its civilian trauma equivalent, given the availability of definitive care further along in the medical chain.[78] In other words, we must restrict our forward operational HSS capabilities solely to those required to preserve life and limb.

Third, we cannot afford to hold stabilized post-surgical patients forward, as doing so will tie the field ambulance down and prevent it from remaining close to the supported forces. We must move beyond our current belief that such patients have to be held immobile for extended periods. This existing paradigm remains solidly entrenched in our emerging joint doctrine, which calls for a 24 to 48 hour post-surgical window prior to further evacuation.[79] Conversely, US experiences in Panama[80] and Iraq[81] have shown that post-surgical casualties can be moved quite quickly, particularly if they are only being evacuated to a supporting Role 3 facility in the rear area. However, the ability to effect early movement of post-surgical patients is critically dependent on a robust air and ground intra-theatre evacuation system.

CONCLUSION

> Overall, the trend during the last 60 years has been for medical organizations to become more deployable, mobile and smaller while retaining significant capabilities with an increased emphasis on forward surgical care and rapid evacuation to an 'appropriate' medical care facility.[82]

Although quite correct in their assessment cited above, Moloff and Denny understate the import of this continuing undercurrent in military medicine. We are now able to bring lifesaving resuscitative surgery far closer to the casualty than ever before. This saves soldiers' lives and will save even more in the future, as we become increasingly capable of reaching those that would otherwise have died on the battlefield or before reaching appropriate forward care.

Our understanding of the physiologic nature of trauma as defined by the "Golden Hour" has never been clearer, and the proven efficacy of far forward resuscitative surgical care continues to be proven in every new major military operation. Given the foregoing, it is not at all surprising to find the increasingly routine employment of Far Forward Surgery at Role 2 units and even below. Despite all of this progress, there remains a perplexing institutional reluctance to assign an organic surgical capability so far down in the HSS chain. This reluctance is all the more puzzling when we consider the future battlespace wherein we will have to provide operational HSS; a battlespace characterized by requirements for mobility, agility, flexibility and responsiveness - the very attributes that define lower level tactical units.

Although the CF has made great strides in developing a credible Role 3 operational HSS capability in the form of 1 Canadian Field Hospital, the existing doctrine and organizational structures that surround this capability will not meet our future battlespace requirements. Indeed, these can only be met when we stop fighting the undercurrent that is pulling casualty care ever forward towards the very battle lines. The time has come to redefine Role 2 operational HSS to include initial resuscitative surgery and to support this redefinition with the establishment of a Far Forward Surgical capability integral to Canadian field ambulances. Doing so will not be without its challenges and will demand certain supporting imperatives, but the advantages to be gained are significant and are critical to positioning operational HSS to support the Army of Tomorrow.

NOTES

1   W.J. Slim, *Defeat Into Victory: Battling Japan in Burma and India*, 1942-1945 (New York: Cooper Square Press, 2000), 18.

2   North Atlantic Treaty Organization (NATO), *Allied Joint Medical Support Doctrine* (Ratification Draft 1), AJP-4.1 (henceforth *AJP-4.10*) (Casteau, Belgium: Supreme Headquarters Allied Powers Europe, 1999), 13.

3   These essays are chapters 1 and 3 in this volume.

4   NATO, *AJP-4.10*, 64.

5   David Salisbury and Allan English, "Prognosis 2020: A Military Medical Strategy for the Canadian Forces," *Canadian Military Journal* 4, no.2 (Summer 2003), 53. A version of this article was originally submitted by Colonel Salisbury in June 2002 as part of the academic requirement for National Strategic Studies Course 4 at the Canadian Forces College (CFC) under the title "Prescription 2020: Considerations for A Military Medical Strategy for the Canadian Forces."

6   J.C. Taylor, "Whither the Field Ambulance? Role 2 Land Health Service Support in the 21st Century Battlespace," paper written for the Advanced Military Studies Course, CFC in 2002, 19. It appears as chapter 3 in this volume.

7   S.E. Henthorne, "Technical Developments in Far Forward Medical Support for the 21st Century Warfighter," *RUSI Journal* 143, no. 5 (October 1998), 41.

8   L.W. Hoff, *The Medical Package for the Objective Force* (Fort Leavenworth, KS: US Army Command and General Staff College Paper, 2002), 6.

9   S. Beaty, "The Revolution in Military Medical Affairs," *Parameters* 27, no. 4 (Winter 1997/1998), 66.

10   S.F. Gouge, *Combat Health Support of the Transformation Force in 2015* (Carlisle Barracks, PA: US Army War College, 2001), 21.

11   A.M. Smith, "Military Medicine: Not the Same as Practicing Medicine in the Military," *Armed Forces and Society* 18, no. 4 (Summer 1992), 579.

12   L.W. Grau and C.J. Gbur, "Mars and Hippocrates in Megapolis: Urban Combat and Medical Support," *US Army Medical Department Journal* no. 8-03-1/2/3 (January/February/March 2003), 21.

13   Gouge, *Combat Health Support of the Transformation Force in 2015*, 21.

14   K. Al-Ali, "Combat Health Support," *Army Logistician* 33, no. 6 (November/December 2001), 40.

15   P.W. Lund, "Medical Support for Future Combat: No More Vietnams," *Naval War College Review* 45, no. 2 (Spring 1992), 88.

16   Beaty, "The Revolution in Military Medical Affairs," 67, 70.

17   J.H.B. Peay, "Correlating Medical Forces Forward," *Joint Force Quarterly* no. 14 (Winter 1996-1997), 72.

18   G. Cecchine, et al., *Army Medical Support to the Army After Next: Issues and Insights from the Medical Technology Workshop*, 1999 (Santa Monica: RAND, 2000), 39.

19   Canada, Department of National Defence, (DND) *Health Services Support to Canadian Forces Operations*, B-GG-005-004/AF-017, draft dated August 2002, (henceforth *HSS to CF Ops*) (Ottawa: DND, 2002), p. 1-5.

20   Ibid., p. 2-1.

21   Gouge, *Combat Health Support of the Transformation Force in 2015*, 6.

22   A.M. Smith, "All Bleeding Stops Eventually," *US Naval Institute Proceedings* 127, no. 11 (November 2001), 68.

23   Taylor, "Whither the Field Ambulance?" 18.

24   T.E. Broyles, *A Comparative Analysis of the Medical Support in the Combat Operations in the Falklands Campaign and the Grenada Expedition* (Fort Leavenworth, KS: US Army Command and General Staff College Paper, 1987), 63.

25   R.D. Handy, "Health Service Support and the Marine Division: A Primer," *Marine Corps Gazette* 77, no. 8 (August 1993), 27.

26   A.M. Smith, "Care Delayed is Care Denied," *Naval War College Review* 52, no. 4 (Autumn 1999), 112.

27   L.W. Grau and T.L. Thomas, "'Soft Log' and Concrete Canyons: Russian Urban Combat Logistics in Grozny," *Marine Corps Gazette* 83, no. 10 (October 1999), 71.

28   J.A. Laterza, *Medical Support of Military Operations on Urban Terrain* (MOUT) (Fort Leavenworth, KS: US Army Command and General Staff College Paper, 2002), 5.

29   Taylor, "Whither the Field Ambulance?" 11.

30   Hoff, "The Medical Package for the Objective Force," 10.

31   DND, *The Interim Army: A Force Employment Discussion Paper* (Ottawa: DND, 2003), p. B-8.

32   A.M. Smith, "Care Delayed is Care Denied," 109.

33   Handy, "Health Service Support and the Marine Division," 25; C.J. Hooton, "Medical Support for the FMF: Far in the Rear, Too Much Gear," *Marine Corps Gazette* 74, no. 4 (April 1990), 52; and Lund, "Medical Support for Future Combat," 88.

34   M. Hewish and J.J. Lok, "Stemming the Flow: Reducing the Rate of Combat Casualties," *Jane's International Defense Review* 32 (December 1999), 9.

35   A.M. Smith, "Adapting is Key for Casualty Care," *US Naval Institute Proceedings* 129, no. 5 (May 2003), 72.

36   Slim, *Defeat Into Victory*, 179.

37   Broyles, *A Comparative Analysis of the Medical Support,* 57.

38   L.W. Grau and M.A. Gress, eds. *The Soviet-Afghan war: How a Superpower Fought and Lost: The Russian General Staff* (Lawrence: University Press of Kansas, 2002), 303.

39   Gouge, *Combat Health Support of the Transformation Force in 2015*, 2, 14.

40   US Army Medical Department (AMEDD), "After Action Reports – Operation Enduring Freedom" and "Initial Lessons Learned Reports – Operation Iraqi Freedom," available from http://www.lessonslearned.amedd.army.mil/, accessed 1 October 2003.

41   DND, *Health Service Support*, B-GL-343-001/FP-000 (Ottawa: DND Canada, 2001), 12. Hereafter *Health Svc Sp.*

42   Ibid., 12.

43   DND, *HSS to CF Ops*, p. 6-6.

44   DND, *Standing Committee on Operational Medicine Review: Phase One Final Report.* (Ottawa: DND Canada, 2001), para 258.

45   US Department of Defense (DoD), *Doctrine for Health Service Support in Joint Operations, Joint Publication 4-02* (Washington: DoD, 2001). Hereafter *US JP 4-02.*

46   US Army, *Medical Platoon Leader's Handbook,* Field Manual 8-10-4 (Washington: DoD, 1990).

47   US Army, *Medical Support in Divisions, Separate Brigades, and the Armored Cavalry Regiment*, Field Manual 8-15 (Washington: DoD, 1972).

48   Hoff, "The Medical Package for the Objective Force," 9.

49   J.T. Need, *Operational Medicine from the Sea: A Revolution in Medical Affairs* (Newport: US Naval War College Paper, 1997), 6.

50   A.M. Smith, "Matching Fleet Medical Readiness to the New Naval Strategy," *US Naval War College Review* 50, no. 1 (Winter 1997), 25-6.

51   NATO, *AJP-4.10*, 14.

52   Ibid., 17.

53   Lieutenant-Colonel C.L. Mitchell, Commanding Officer 1 Canadian Field Hospital, e-mail to author, 1 October 2003.

54   Gouge, *Combat Health Support of the Transformation Force in 2015*, 23.

55   DND, *Health Svc Sp*, 93.

56   DND, *HSS to CF Ops*, p. 6-27.

57   Ibid.

58   Hewish and Lok, "Stemming the Flow," 47.

59   Henthorne, "Technical Developments in Far Forward Medical Support for the 21st Century Warfighter," 41-2.

60   Laterza, *Medical Support of Military Operations on Urban Terrain* (MOUT), 3.

61   Cecchine, et al., *Army Medical Support to the Army After Next*, 44.

62   Lieutenant-Colonel K. Moore, DAPVB 3 NDHQ Ottawa, e-mail correspondence with Colonel A.C. Patch, 21 October 2003.

63   Salisbury and English, "Prognosis 2020," 49.

64   US AMEDD, "Initial Lessons Learned Reports – Operation Iraqi Freedom."

65   D.R. Porr, *To Be There, To Be Ready and To Save Lives* (Carlisle Barracks, PA: US Army War College Paper, 1993), 11.

66   US AMEDD, "82nd Forward Support Battalion After Action Report – Operation Enduring Freedom," para 3.i. Available from http://www.lessonslearned.amedd.army.mil/, accessed 1 October 2003.

67   *US JP 4-02*, II-1.

68   A.L. Moloff and S. Denny, "The Contingency Medical Force: Chronic Challenge, New Solutions," US Army Report 212th MASH, 1999. Available from http://secure-ll.amedd.army.mil/Reports/CMFartide.htm, accessed 1 October 2003.

69   Allan D. English, "Leadership and Operational Stress in the Canadian Forces," *Canadian Military Journal* 1, no. 2 (Autumn, 2000), 36.

70   A.M Smith, "Joint Medical Support: Are We Asleep at the Switch?" *Joint Force Quarterly*, no. 8 (Summer 1995), 104.

71   Moloff and Denny, "The Contingency Medical Force," 2.

72   US AMEDD, "102nd Forward Surgical Team After Action Report – Operation Enduring Freedom," section I, para 1. Available from http://www.lessonslearned.amedd.army.mil/, accessed 1 October 2003.

73   DND, *Shaping the Future of the Canadian Forces: A Strategy for 2020* (Ottawa: DND, 1999).

74   DND, *Advancing With Purpose: The Army Strategy* (Ottawa: DND, 2002).

75   DND, *HSS to CF Ops*, p. 2-8.

76   Smith, "Military Medicine," 585.

77   Hooton, "Medical Support for the FMF," 51.

78   Porr, *To Be There, To Be Ready and To Save Lives*, 9.

79   DND, *HSS to CF Ops*, p. 3-9.

80   P.K. Carlton, "New Millennium, New Mind-Set: The Air Force Medical Service in the Air Expeditionary Era," *Aerospace Power Journal* 15, no. 4 (Winter, 2001), 11.

81   US AMEDD, "Initial Lessons Learned Reports – Operation Iraqi Freedom."

82   Moloff and Denny, "The Contingency Medical Force," 2.

CHAPTER 5

HEALTH SERVICES SUPPORT IN THE 21ST CENTURY: THE NEED TO REPLACE FIELD AMBULANCES WITH TAILORED MODULAR CAPABILITIES

Lieutenant-Colonel C.L. Mitchell

INTRODUCTION

The Canadian Forces (CF) is undergoing a significant transformation process to conduct operations in the non-linear, non-contiguous future battlespace. CF transformation and the future battlespace will shape how combat service support (CSS) is organized and provided. Therefore, CSS organizations cannot afford to maintain an attachment to past CSS doctrine and structures, as they will not be helpful in future operations. To meet the emerging support challenges of 21st century military operations, the Canadian Forces Health Services (CFHS) has drafted Health Service Support (HSS) doctrine that aligns HSS along modular, building block capabilities, rather than unit structures. However, current HSS field ambulances are structured to support former doctrine based on a linear battlefield. If field ambulances are not restructured along modular capabilities, then there is a danger that wounded soldiers may not receive surgical intervention in a timely manner. Indeed, lessons learned from military medical experiences of US and UK medical facilities in Iraq can provide valuable assistance for modifying CFHS operational support structures along modular capabilities. By replacing existing field ambulances structures with modular capabilities tailored to suit the operation, CFHS will be better able to meet the land component HSS requirements of future battlespaces.

This chapter will restrict its discussion to the provision of HSS to land operations. It will provide the background perspective on the debate over the continued utility of field ambulances as they currently exist, as well as provide the current CF strategic concepts that underpin emerging CFHS doctrine. It will review the current health doctrine of Canadian, US and UK militaries for similarities in the doctrinal provision of HSS, especially in the areas of modular capability.   Lessons learned and suggested capability modifications in after action reviews by our allies during recent operations will highlight how practice varies from doctrine. This analysis is offered as food for thought for Canadian HSS planners as they task tailor HSS for Canadian operations, and will discuss concerns the HSS community has in supporting the future battlespace. Finally, this chapter will outline the potential impact HSS can have on the operational level in tradeoffs between mobility and provision of surgical support that may be ameliorated by restructuring field ambulances into modular facilities.

BACKGROUND - THE DEBATE

Discussion regarding the future employment and utility of Canadian field ambulances has been ongoing for a number of years.   In 1997, Major G. Richardson initiated early commentary on the continued role of field ambulances in provision of medical support to the army. Richardson recommended the removal of brigade field ambulances, as their capabilities can be provided by other organizations. To provide medical support to brigades, Richardson recommended that Unit Medical Stations (UMS) be fully manned and equipped to alleviate the need for augmentation from field ambulances.   Additionally, Richardson argued that field ambulances have no legitimate role in Operations Other Than War (OOTW), and that the robust ground evacuation capabilities field ambulances can bring to mid-intensity operations could be provided by the medical Reserve units. Furthermore, she asserted that disbanding of the field ambulances could provide valuable personnel offsets to augment Role 1 and 3 units, while allowing medical personnel to be posted to units that would give them a greater opportunity to regularly practice their medical skills.[1]

More recently, the continued existence of field ambulances in their current structure was once again challenged when the ability of existing CF Health Services organizations to support emerging military operational trends, future military health clients, future casualty trends and the potential of new technology on medicine in battle was considered.   Salisbury and English argued that these factors have so significantly changed the HSS operating environment that "This will bring into question the existence and role of the Field Ambulance, as it currently exists." They go on to further amplify that building-block modules may represent the best way ahead as, "Mass casualties are unlikely, and thus the deployment of the entire field hospital as it currently exists is unlikely, and modules of the field hospital similar to the current Advanced Surgical Centres (ASCs) will become the norm."[2] Taylor continued this discussion, recommending the retention of the current capabilities of the Field Ambulance along with its task-tailored augmentation by a resuscitative surgical capability, and the addition of a dedicated aeromedical evacuation capability.[3] Subsequently, Weger went on to recommend the establishment of an integral far-forward surgical capability within CF Field Ambulances.[4]

THE IMPACT OF DOCTRINE

The Concepts supporting CFHS Doctrine. The CF Strategic Operating Concept (SOC) provides an "overarching conceptual framework for designing the CF of the future," as a key tenet for shaping CF transformation. Its focus is on planning for events five to 15 years from now. The CF SOC has drawn a picture of the current and future security environments that acknowledge the impact of globalization, failing states, multidimensional battlespace, stressors in littoral regions and unconventional threats upon the organization and capability of the CF. The SOC identifies the need for the CF to have the capacity to operate in mid-intensity combat operations, stating that a force able to operate in combat can transition to lower intensity operations with more ease than forces transitioning the other way. The SOC also warns that threats to Canada will require a CF able to provide a "multidisciplinary approach" to meet those threats.[5]

To address support, sustainment and mobility issues, the SOC provides specific direction on expected Department of Defence and CF capabilities. The SOC direction specifically addressing health capabilities requires the following: "A force health protection capability that covers the full range of health threats and force enablers from prevention and health promotion through immediate life and limb saving capability, to evacuation and rehabilitation to return personnel to duty."[6]

By 2012, it is anticipated that the CF will have acquired operational reach, i.e., the capacity to operate away from a national support base for extended periods of time. Doctrinally, this will be achieved through the acquisition of more strategic lift capability, enhanced deployment enablers, diplomatic arrangements for overflight clearances, multinational reception and staging cooperation, logistic agreements and material pre-positioning. Synchronization of logistics support activities from strategic through operational and tactical levels will be achieved through a shared CF Common Operating Picture (CF COP) and provided by the National Military Support Capability (NMSC).[7] The NMSC project is currently ongoing and is expected upon rollout to optimize CF support to deployed operations in joint and coalition operations. In the context of CF transformation, the future of the NMSC project is presently unknown, but the NMSC project does provide an existing, valuable model for deployed operational support.

CFHS has been involved with the NMSC project from its inception, as the limited HSS resources available to place in theatre are expected to provide HSS to joint operations. From CFHS's perspective, NMSC optimizes the seamless sustainment capability expected by deployed commanders. The NMSC Concept of Operations has broken the functions and tasks for deployed operations down to the appropriate environmental commands for their action. CFHS's provision of HSS support to an operational deployment, under command of the Joint Support Group Headquarters (JSGHQ), will be to provide from Role 1 to Role 3 HSS capability through a Joint Health Support Unit (JHSU) to support the joint troops.[8] This facility is intended to be collocated in the same camp as the JSGHQ although the operational situation may dictate a different solution on deployment. The camp layout is based on a hub-and-spoke concept, with the relatively immobile support organizations inside the joint support camp. This particular layout addresses current CF support in a non-linear, non-contiguous theatre, which allows patrols to go out in the area and return to a relatively secure, defended area. This concept may not be applicable if operations shift from hub-and-spoke operations to mobility operations.

The JHSU is intended to deploy with its own integral support, less vehicle technicians and food services personnel. In consultations with the CFHS Working Group, the Joint Workshop and Joint Food Services Working Groups agreed to allocate personnel to provide services to the JHSU in exchange for personnel offsets to meet the additional JHSU demands.[9]

In structure, role, and organization, the JHSU resembles an Advanced Surgical Center (ASC), a sub-unit of 1 Canadian Field Hospital. Both organizations are built upon the following eight modules: 1) a command and control module, 2) an integral Role 1 and 2[10] modular capability for HSS support to area troops, 3) a reception and resuscitation module, 4) a surgical and sterilization module, 5) a pharmacy services module, 6) a diagnostics and therapeutics module, 7) patient ward modules and 8) a support platoon. Neither the ASC or JHSU organization has integral ambulance assets; however, both organizations can have evacuation modules placed under control or under command from higher formations for medical evacuation. While the holding capacity of either structure will be tailored to suit the mission and theatre holding policies, ASCs are organized to have one 5-bed critical care ward and one 10-bed intermediate care ward.[11] ASCs must meet the following five essential operational criteria: 1) be capable of accepting patients within three hours and conducting surgery within five hours of arrival in location; 2) be self-sufficient at first line; 3) be equipped to provide initial surgery, patient care and holding in climatic conditions where CF formations can be deployed; 4) be capable of deploying in terrain similar to those formations being supported; 5) have adequate protection characteristics, including the capability of deploying patient treatment areas in or outside buildings and low noise, infra-red and electronic emission signatures.[12] The JHSU is expected to meet the same operational criteria as an ASC.

ASCs have been consistently deployed on CF operations since the initial deployment of an ASC from 1 Canadian Field Hospital into the Former Republic of Yugoslavia in 1991. The present Canadian HSS facility for Operation ATHENA in Kabul is identified as a NATO Role 2+,[13] as it can provide initial life-saving surgical support in theatre. It contains an evacuation module from field ambulances and a surgical module from 1 Canadian Field Hospital. The planned HSS facility slated for Operation ATHENA in Kandahar (February 2006) will be a Role 3 facility, similar to an ASC in capability, with an additional robust evacuation module, as it is intended to provide Role 3 HSS support to the multinational brigade as well as Canadian soldiers.

Review of Canadian, US and UK Doctrine. A review of Canadian, US and UK HSS doctrine reveals that all three countries share common operating philosophies and have organized their HSS in a similar fashion to meet operational demands. There is some variance in terminology, however. While Canadian and UK doctrine use the term "role" to describe medical support, US doctrine uses the term "echelon."

Canadian HSS Doctrine. CFHS doctrine is based on roles of support. Roles of HSS support are based on clinical capabilities required within the operational environment and on the requirement to provide Force Health Protection. Clinical capabilities refer to the progressive examination, treatment, evacuation and hospitalization of sick and injured personnel.[14] At point of wounding, casualties will receive first aid and emergency medical treatment at the Role 1 facility – a Unit Medical Station – and will be triaged and stabilized prior to evacuation to the next role of care, if needed. At Role 2 facilities – the Brigade Medical Station – rapid evacuation of stabilized casualties is provided while they are enroute to sustaining care. Emergency lifesaving resuscitation may be performed at Role 2 facilities, but they have very limited holding capability. Those casualties who require a longer recovery time to return to duty in excess of the unit holding policy will be evacuated rearward. Role 3 facilities – Advanced Surgical Centers and field hospitals – emphasize resuscitation, initial wound surgery, pre- and post- operative care, diagnostic services (laboratory and x-ray), blood storage, intermediate and critical care wards, and limited internal medicine and psychiatric services. Role 4 facilities are normally out of theatre definitive care hospitals that can provide a full range of surgery, rehabilitation, storage of national HSS stocks and major repair/replacement of HSS equipment. HSS facilities in theatre can be augmented, to a limited degree, with some of the capabilities from the role above it.

US Army Medical Echelons of Support. US Health Services Support doctrine in joint operations is based on conserving the fighting strength of land, sea, air and special operations forces through minimizing the effects of wounds and disease on unit effectiveness, readiness and morale. US HSS is based on five echelons of care, with each echelon providing increasingly sophisticated interventions. Maintaining HSS proximity to supported troops allows HSS facilities to treat casualties as close to combat operations as the tactical situation permits and to evacuate casualties rearward only as far as the severity of their wounds dictate.

At Echelon I, casualties receive care at the unit level, including self and buddy aid, examination and emergency lifesaving measures. In addition, this echelon may also have an aid station with a physician or physician assistant (PA). At Echelon II, a casualty will receive care from a team of physicians or PAs, and care at this echelon includes basic resuscitation and stabilization. It may also include surgical capability, basic laboratory, limited x-ray, pharmacy and a temporary holding capability. At Echelon III, resuscitation, initial surgery and post-operative treatment is provided. A casualty may receive here the first stage of comprehensive surgical treatment intended to restore him or her to functional health. Hospital ships are used to provide some Echelon III medical care.[15] Echelon IV care provides definitive therapy for casualties and may provide a recovery phase for those who are expected to return to duty within the theatre evacuation policy. Echelon V care is convalescent and rehabilitative care normally provided by military, civilian or Department of Veterans Affairs hospitals in United States. Care here is intended to restore patients to functional health with the objective of returning to duty or a useful life upon release.

The US Army Medical Department (AMEDD) has taken advantage of technological gains in field medical capabilities to meet current operational requirements. To address the need of far forward medical care, Forward Surgical Team (FST) modules have been successfully trialed in multiple operations. FSTs are relatively small and flexible units that can complete approximately ten surgeries per day and the post-operative care associated with those surgeries until patients can be evacuated rearward for more definitive care. FSTs can deploy in the area of a manoeuvre brigade or armoured cavalry regiment and typically have a staff of 20 members organized into four functional areas: triage-trauma, surgery, post-surgical recovery and administration/operations. With two operating tables, each FST can provide initial surgery and up to six hours of post-operative care for up to eight patients at a time. Surgical interventions include major chest and abdominal wounds, hemorrhage, severe shock, airway and respiratory distress, amputations, major organ fractures, crush injuries and acute deteriorating consciousness from closed head wounds.[16] FSTs are not mobile while surgery is ongoing and patients are recovering post-operatively prior to medical evacuation rearward.

UK Roles of Medical Support. British Army Medical Services (AMS) doctrine has been adapted, since the first Gulf War in 1991, from supporting a Cold War scenario to supporting military operations that are more expeditionary in nature. Additionally, wherever possible, service personnel will be offered a standard of health care equal to that they would expect to receive in the UK during peacetime. As a consequence, UK defence chiefs have been willing to expend significantly more resources on managing critically ill or injured casualties who would have, in past, been managed as expectant (i.e., unlikely to survive) cases in Cold War scenarios.[17]

British Army medical doctrine is built upon a chain of medical care organized into Roles and extending from point of wounding to definitive rehabilitative medical care in the UK, with a focus on maintaining the fighting strength of the Army.[18] At point of wounding, a casualty receives "buddy" aid or self-aid and then progresses to a Regimental Aid Post (Role 1) for resuscitation, if required. At the aid post, a medical doctor assesses the casualty and Battlefield Advanced Trauma Life Support (BATLS) is initiated, when necessary. From the aid post, the casualty is evacuated to a medical dressing station (Role 2) that may be augmented with a surgical capability (Role 2+). Surgery at this facility is only initiated to ensure the casualty will survive further evacuation rearward to the field hospital (Role 3). At the field hospital, definitive surgical care is provided and the casualty is prepared for repatriation to a rehabilitation facility (Role 4) in the UK. Throughout the chain of evacuation, the casualty is constantly monitored to address any life threatening symptoms, and priority of evacuation is given to the most seriously wounded casualties. UK medical doctrine acknowledges the tension between needed mobility and clinical capability. The more clinically capable a hospital, the less mobile it becomes; conversely, the lighter and smaller a facility, the better it can keep up with manoeuvre elements. The cost, however, of increased mobility is borne in compromising clinical outcomes and care environments.[19]

IMPROVING CASUALTY SURVIVABILITY

In medical parlance, increased likelihood of wounded soldiers surviving their injuries is based upon the construct of the "Golden Hour." The term identifies the importance of providing definitive protocols in rapid medical assessment and resuscitative care, including surgery, as critical to patient survival and, as such, is considered to be a benchmark standard in present trauma management.[20] It is described in Advanced Trauma Life Support (ATLS) protocols as the period in which rapid medical assessment and resuscitation is required,[21] in order to improve the likelihood of casualty survival. There is ongoing learned discussion regarding the efficacy of applying this terminology to combat casualties, as it was initially coined to describe the resuscitation timings required for victims of blunt-trauma injury and does not truly reflect the significantly more urgent care requirements of combat casualties with penetrating trauma.[22] For the purpose of this chapter, highlighting the discussion on the use of this terminology is intended to draw the reader's attention to the urgent requirement for combat casualties to receive surgical care as soon as possible after wounding, and as close to the "Golden Hour" timing as possible.

Combat casualties can be described using a bi-modal distribution of mortality. According to this model, approximately 90 percent of combat deaths occur within five minutes of wounding, including those combat casualties who die of severe wounds within seconds of injury.[23] Of those who survive past that time, an additional 15 percent of deaths occur within 30 minutes of wounding. Between thirty minutes and six hours post-wounding, 5 to 20 percent of casualties will die, with half of those deaths occurring in the first two hours after wounding. Gouge advises that, unless early treatment for shock and removal of any penetrating infectious material is initiated, sepsis and multi-organ failure will occur, leading to 60 percent mortality rates.[24] Unless casualties receive ATLS within the first hour, many will not survive long enough to reach surgical facilities. Prompt evacuation of those casualties with serious wounds is vital; otherwise, those soldiers are likely to die between 30 minutes and six hours after injury. The importance of casualties receiving speedy access to definitive treatment is acknowledged in CF doctrine:

> The shock-producing affect of blood loss from injury is worsened by other fluid depletion, such as from significant burns, vomit-ing, diarrhea, perspiration, or limited fluid intake. For those with very severe shock, the Advanced Trauma Life Support (ATLS) principle of the 'golden hour' applies.[25]

CF doctrine goes on to say that "life/limb-saving clinical intervention must be provided as soon as possible, ideally within the first hour, but completed not later than six hours following onset of life/limb-threatening injury."[26] Based on this doctrine, an argument can be made for placing surgical capability as far forward as is practicable: if surgery can be performed within the "Golden Hour," soldiers' lives can be saved; if it is not, then death will be the most likely result.

The role of efficient and timely medical evacuation from point of wounding to a medical facility able to deal with the nature of the injury is essential in improving patient survival. Medical evacuation (MEDEVAC) can be conducted using ground or air ambulance assets and should not transport the casualty rearward of the most forward treatment facility with the capability to treat that casualty's level of injury. The nature of the battlespace will determine the degree to which the total medical footprint can be reduced in theatre. Further, the capability to stabilize casualties and rapidly evacuate them out of theatre needs to be balanced with the requirement to have a degree of hospitalization capability in theatre. As technological advances have increased the enemy's ability to strike anywhere in friendly territory, the likely extension of evacuation distances to offset this threat cannot be discounted. Extended evacuation distances reduce patient survivability and also render evacuation assets more vulnerable to enemy fire.[27]

The helicopter has proven itself to be a reliable platform for medical evaluation in past conflicts, and its ability to speedily transport wounded to surgical facilities has ensured that wounded are more likely to reach surgical facilities within the "Golden Hour." The helicopter's ability to transport wounded to a medical facility more quickly than can be provided by ground evacuation assets has increased the flexibility of the medical plan in past operations. The increased reliance on aeromedical evacuation (AME) caused two distinct changes to combat medical support. As this reliance brought air evacuation to the forward areas, medicine became increasingly dependent upon it to move casualties. Additionally, entire generations of medical personnel became increasingly comfortable with reducing the mobility of medical units and with retaining comprehensive medical support in the rear. An evacuation plan that utilizes helicopter and AME resources assumes that friendly forces will have air superiority, enabling air medevac to take place when and where it is needed.[28]

With US medical evacuation in past conflicts, this has been reality; however, current and future operating environments contain the threat to aircraft from shoulder-fired missiles. These weapons have advanced lethality and accuracy, and their proliferation has increased their availability to enemy forces. Ongoing discussion suggests the modern and future battlespace may be too lethal to support continued reliance upon air evacuation of wounded, and the continued survivability of helicopters in that environment is not assured. Further, the present heavy reliance upon air evacuation of casualties by helicopter may need to be revisited to address the support required in future operations.[29]

RECENT US AND UK OPERATIONAL MEDICAL EXPERIENCES

US Medical Lessons Learned from Operation Iraqi Freedom. American after action reports (AAR) suggested that the overall size of Combat Support Hospitals (CSH) was too large and recommended that CSH facilities should be divided into two independent surgical facilities, based upon the experiences of dividing the 21st CSH and given the casualty workloads of the split facility in two locations. The 21st CSH North had 44 beds and 21st CSH South had 84 beds. Generally, the peak capacity at CSH North was, on average, 30 patients, and with the capacity to evacuate post-surgical patients, expectations were that mass casualty situations could be met by the split units.

AAR also highlighted deployment issues regarding required coordination to ensure engineer support for ground preparation prior to the arrival of the CSH. Further, the reports identified an ongoing need to have integral lift capability within CSHs, while acknowledging the efficacy of Corps assets such as the Rough Terrain Cargo Handlers to move the CSH's containers once a site had been selected. Having no integral lift made CSHs reliant upon external lift assets held at US Army Corps level, and usually these assets are not made available easily during the early phases of an operation. The AAR also identified pieces of equipment within the CSH that worked well, as well as diagnostic equipment (e.g., CT scanner and microbiology capability) that needed to be added to the standard operating equipment of a CSH.[30] Additionally, AMEDD is currently designing lighter, more efficient shelters to accommodate field hospitals and is investigating the application of telemedicine with lightweight portable diagnostic equipment for deployments.[31]

These lessons are relevant to the discussion of modular capability as the US experiences suggest that smaller modules can meet the surgical demands of current operations. Their lack of internal lift and its impact on the mobility of the unit is a reminder to Canadian HSS planners to consider maintaining a service support module as part of the new HSS model, depending on the anticipated mobility of the CF operation.

UK Medical Lessons Learned from Operation TELIC. During Operation TELIC, UK land forces were supported by two field hospitals, one located in Kuwait and the second hospital, 202 Field Hospital, at the abandoned Iraqi Air Force base at Shaibah, Iraq. 202 Field Hospital had no integral lift and relied upon the Joint Forces Logistics Brigade to move it into location. The field hospital was moved in 67 container carriers and the containers were dropped into the general location. With its integral container handling capability, the hospital quickly opened 25 beds and two operating rooms (ORs) to meet anticipated initial casualties, and then set up the remainder of the operating rooms, to a total of seven ORs. The hospital did not set up its complete 200-bed capability, as patients tended to be speedily airlifted out of theatre to Kuwait or onward to the UK. The field hospital remained more forward of the Role 2 medical assets of 7ᵗʰ Armoured Brigade, rendering this Role 2 capability redundant. Despite the presence of combat surgical teams attached to the Role 2 facilities, the majority of wounded were evacuated straight back to the Role 3 facility by either armoured ambulance or helicopters.[32] Generally, casualties were received at the field hospital within 20 minutes of wounding when evacuated by helicopter and within one hour by road ambulance.

202 Field Hospital admitted 1,366 patients during the warfighting phase of Operation TELIC (17 March - 30 April 2003). The majority of admissions were ballistic trauma, gunshot wounds or shrapnel and then burns. After the conclusion of the warfighting phase (1 May - 20 July 2003), the majority of medical admissions shifted from ballistic trauma and burns to heat injuries and blunt trauma injuries from road accidents.[33]

Security of medical facilities is always of concern to operational planners. In the case of a Role 3 Field Hospital, the footprint, size, complex integral systems within the facility and patient requirements are such that the facility is not readily mobile and is not intended to defend itself. 202 (UK) Field Hospital in Shaibah was protected by layered defences: by its physical location on the vast Shaibah Airfield, by the presence of a dedicated Quick Reaction Force (QRF), and by other joint troops on the airfield and a point defence missile system.[34]

Operation TELIC provided operational medical planners with an opportunity to learn valuable lessons and review the planning assumptions used in estimating medical support to operations. Basing the medical estimate on the medical experiences of Operation Agricola (Kosovo 1999), medical planners underestimated the intensity of the expected workload for Operation TELIC in that the proportion of intubated and ventilated patients was significantly higher than expected (44.5 percent). Specifically, planners did not anticipate that many patients would require a significant period of post-operative ventilation while they were undergoing resuscitation. The major difference in patient admissions between 202 Field Hospital and hospitals with past peace support operations was in the greater number of ballistic trauma patients filling the Intensive Care Units.

Additionally, there were medical support requirements that needed to be addressed. It was impossible to maintain a reasonable ambient air temperature in the tented facility during the heat of the day and, as a consequence, the body temperature of burn patients became critically high. During sandstorms, the facility became extremely dusty and staff was forced to stop ventilator testing to reduce sand accumulations in the equipment. Noise was a constant problem as well: air conditioners and generators affected the quality of clinical examinations. Medical support to Operation TELIC highlighted the requirement for planners to address an important logistical issue: facilities may not be able to rapidly evacuate their casualties, and some post-surgical complications may need to be managed in theatre, despite the doctrinal focus of rapid evacuation out of theatre.[35]

Lessons learned from the UK experience demonstrated the importance of placing Role 3 surgical support forward with appropriate security arrangements, as this facility was heavy to lift. As in the US case, UK field hospitals lack integral lift and must rely on joint logistics units to move them. The presence of the Role 3 facility rendered the Role 2 facility redundant, as wounded could be speedily evacuated to the Role 3 facility. In this instance, the facility was very large and the number of casualties it handled during the operation indicated that the size of this facility was appropriate to the circumstances. From the UK experience, Canadian HSS planners can draw three important lessons. First, during the medical planning process, they must seriously consider including integral lift modules in the development of medical facility. Second, they need to keep in mind that limiting the sophistication of the medical facility to "bare bones" will exacerbate heat, dust and sterility concerns to the detriment of the wounded. And third, they must consider the need for additional security requirements at the facilities, depending on their mobility.

SUPPORTING THE FUTURE BATTLESPACE

If past CF military doctrine described a two-dimensional battlefield with opposing forces facing off against each other, what will future combat and combat service support look like? Current expectations have shifted to acknowledge the increasing likelihood that our forces will be facing asymmetric combat threats in a non-linear, non-contiguous battlespace. Additionally, the rising prevalence and complexity of urban operations will shape the way combat service support, including HS support, is delivered.[36] Further, military forces of the 21st century must be prepared to operate in an urban environment and to meet that challenge from a positive perspective, not a defeatist attitude.[37] The asymmetric threats facing deployed forces will remain a concern in future operations.

Asymmetric warfare can be described as those means used by adversaries to focus their attack on an opposing military's organizational weaknesses while avoiding their opponents' conventional strengths. In the modern context, asymmetric threats target unexpected vulnerabilities, resulting in heightened surprise and a lengthened response cycle. These actions cause unacceptable friendly force losses and prevent a decisive victory for friendly forces, while asymmetric forces can disguise their intent, strategy and capabilities. Additionally, they may choose to avoid having attacks attributed to them, with a result of achieving their objective and avoiding retaliatory response.[38] The nature of asymmetric warfare is inherently unpredictable and asymmetries between opposing forces of will, technology, organization and time can exist at strategic, operational and tactical levels.[39]

Certainly, the Russian experiences in the urban battle for Grozny (January-February 1995) can provide a useful perspective on the difficulty of providing HSS in a non-linear, non-contiguous battlespace. Their experience indicates that future battles may be conducted different-ly than in past. Russian Army medical support was well planned and special medical treatment detachments were trained prior to the attack on Grozny. The Russians used their normal system of mainly ground medical evacuation, not anticipating that they would be facing a different enemy in the urban operations of Grozny. The wounded were first evacuated by armoured ambulances to a medical aid post and then evacuated rearward by medical helicopter to military hospitals. Chechen fighters deliberately targeted medical assets and facilities, disrupting medical support during operations. Forward medical posts and hospitals needed to be dug in or placed in basements to limit the impact of Chechen shelling on medical facilities. After several medical evacuation helicopters and aircraft were shot down, forward air evacuation was not frequently utilized. As a consequence, statistics of wounded to killed ratios became skewed to 4:1 from the expected 2:1 ratio, because most of those wounded who died were unable to be treated or evacuated.[40] Snipers targeted medical personnel, and Russian wounded frequently could only be evacuated under cover of darkness. A ruthless enemy who shot down AME helicopters and bombed field hospitals in violation of the Geneva Conventions took actions that the Russians either could not or would not contemplate.

This concern is also reflected in Smith's discussion on the nature of future operations and how medical support may be affected:

> For medical evacuation, the helicopter has been an ideal vehicle, but future guided munitions may limit its effectiveness. Instead of medical extractions in minutes, we may have to return to the hand litter, wheeled vehicles, or "walking" casualties. It may take hours or even days for casualties to reach forward hospitals for primary surgical care, resulting in higher fatality rates among those with head, chest and abdominal injuries.[41]

HSS CONCERNS WITH SUPPORTING THE FUTURE BATTLESPACE

Medical planners must wrestle with the most effective way to provide HSS to forces in non-linear, non-contiguous battlespaces, especially when those operations may be engaging enemy forces willing to target HSS facilities and personnel to disrupt friendly forces and gain the advantage of surprise. There are dynamic tensions amongst mobility and definitive treatment, the location of surgical capabilities and the proper skill set of medical personnel when considering medical support in future operations. These tactical issues can have a significant impact on the operational level, as the mobility and capability of HSS facilities may limit an operational commander's plan.

A key question in this debate is - how mobile can a medical facility reasonably expect to be? A rapidly changing, non-contiguous battlespace presents a unique challenge to the provision of HSS, as lines of communication and logistic routes can be rendered vulnerable and evacuation routes can be rendered insecure. If evacuation routes are lost, then existing evacuation assets are in danger of becoming overwhelmed, even in the absence of mass casualty situations. In response to this variable, HSS planners can place medical treatment capability, including surgical support, more forward.[42] The decision to place capability forward is based on the current doctrinal construct of evacuating only relatively stable patients rearward. However, moving treatment forward raises the dynamic tension between increased treatment capability and reduced mobility and raises the specter of evacuating less stable patients rearward in order to address casualty treatment within the "Golden Hour." Also, placing surgical capability forward may lead to surgeons in those forward locations attempting surgeries that are better initiated at a more comprehensive rearward facility. While the enthusiasm of those forward surgeons is commendable, the unintended secondary outcome can involve unnecessary patient morbidity or mortality.

Mobility is a characteristic that medical facilities wish to achieve to remain close to the units they are supporting and be in accordance the operational commander's plan, but mobility must be balanced against the specific requirements of patient treatment. AMEDD is currently looking to field even more mobile shelters for forward surgical treatment, but, in reality, medical facilities are mobile only until they receive casualties. Then mobility becomes moot. Physicians with combat surgical experience have identified that a reasonable planning figure for surgery is a duration of approximately two and one-half hours.[43] Also, post surgical recovery and stabilization for further rearward evacuation of casualties will limit any mobility of medical units until those patients can be cleared from the facility.

Given the ongoing concern with the safety of evacuation vehicles during future operations, forward surgical care must be considered as a viable option, otherwise HSS support in the future battlespace may not be possible. The challenge in providing far forward surgical care is that without robust evacuation assets, the facility is in danger of being overwhelmed as soon as all operating tables are filled and casualties continue to arrive. The needs of those casualties undergoing surgery are being met but those awaiting surgery might have been better off being evacuated rearward by the time the surgical team gets to them.[44] In considering this situation, a panel of physicians recommended that AMEDD investigate an opportunity to combine evacuation and treatment platforms to provide high volume, therapeutic care while enroute to rearward facilities. They felt that this technological advance would allow surgery to be initiated enroute on relatively unstable patients as a way to provide surgical care within the "Golden Hour." The panel felt this might be a reasonable opportunity to explore, provided evacuation platforms can be developed to provide therapeutic care in a relatively stable environment.[45] Until these platforms can be developed and trialed, it is important for medical planners not to assume away these issues by relying on next generation technology that is currently unavailable.

During a seminar on medical support to the Army After Next, discussion ensued regarding the efficacy of non-definitive battlefield care. A study comparing morbidity and mortality outcomes of casualties provided with battlefield treatment and those who did not receive treatment indicated that non-definitive (i.e., non-surgical) treatment was not an indicator of a positive outcome. Rather, the important factor seemed to be speedy access to definitive care, such as that provided by trauma surgery.[46]

MODULAR CAPABILITIES PROVIDE BEST HSS OPTIONS

The discussion to this point has laid the groundwork for the argument that, given the likelihood that the most important factor in patient survivability is speedy access to trauma surgery, the current field ambulance structures should be replaced with modularized capabilities that include surgical modules. This section will discuss the doctrinal, mobility and holding capabilities based on allied experiences that support this argument.

Review of allied doctrine indicates that the US, UK and Canada all have very similar doctrine based on appropriate treatment at progressively more sophisticated medical or HSS facilities as the casualty is evacuated rearward. All countries' doctrine indicates that casualties should go no further rearward than the treatment facility necessary to address their wounds. HSS and medical doctrine are focused on maintaining the fighting fitness of forces and, once wounded, the organization focuses on providing appropriate care to casualties with the intent of returning them to battle or repatriating them out of theatre for definitive rehabilitative care.

Interestingly, US AAR suggests that the CSH may be too big for current and future operations, as they are relatively less mobile and have excess patient capacity. The recommendation of the AAR, to divide CSH capability in half, speaks to the possibility of modularization of CSH assets in future operations. While the modularized CSH would have a larger holding capacity than an ASC, it shares similar capabilities.

US AAR and UK feedback also voiced concerns that CSH and UK field hospitals do not have integral lift and consequently are reliant upon higher organizations to provide it. The difficulty with this arrangement is that medical facilities may require it at the same time as other supported organizations and compete with them for scarce lift resources. By modularizing HSS, medical facilities can add an integral lift and support module to move delicate medical equipment and temperature-sensitive drugs, reagents and equipment. A modular medical facility with similar capabilities to an ASC can be efficiently moved with six 50-foot trailers.

The UK medical experience during Operation TELIC identified several key issues that indicate that field ambulances would be less than effective in current operations. Despite the presence of Role 2 facilities supporting 7th Armoured Brigade, casualties were evacuated directly from Role 1 facilities to the Role 3 hospitals, bypassing the Role 2 facilities in favour of a facility that could provide more definitive care. UK Role 3 facilities struck a balance between mobility and bringing equipment that could have improved patient diagnosis and comfort. For example, the noise, dust, and high internal temperatures experienced inside the Role 3 tent lines could have been alleviated with increased air-conditioning capability and containerized facilities; however, including these capabilities would have increased lift requirements and decreased mobility. However, the UK field hospitals did not move, as they were sited forward of 7th Armoured Brigade Role 2 facilities and were located in a well-defended area. Similarly, the NMSC JSG facilities, including the JHSU, are intended to remain in a defended location in support of hub-and-spoke operations. This solution may be a reasonable response to asymmetric threats, given current CF equipment holdings. Operational planners must resist the desire to wish away the limitations inherent in current equipment realities with futuristic, untried technology that may or may not mitigate the issue at hand, and may bring its own unanticipated problems to the operation.

The ability to hold casualties post-operatively is possible in modular facilities with capabilities based on ASCs and/or Role 3 facilities because they have the integral medical support equipment to monitor patients in recovery wards. Current field ambulances cannot hold post-operative patients, as they do not have that capability. Placing surgical, diagnostics, and holding capabilities in an existing field ambulance change its structure into one similar to an ASC, and renders it less mobile. The Russian experience in Grozny, in response to the Chechen sniping at medical personnel, bombing of their medical facilities and destruction of medical evacuation assets, was to dig in medical facilities. They did not attempt to make their medical facilities more mobile in that environment because the facilities could either move or provide treatment but could not do both in the presence of an enemy that actively engaged non-combatants. Additionally, both Smith[47] and Roberts et al.[48] warn that facilities need to have a robust holding capability and that some post surgical complications may need to be managed in theatre. Despite the doctrinal requirement of evacuation rearward and out of theatre as required, the present reliance upon aircraft for medical evacuation may reveal a weakness to be exploited by the enemy, as was the Russian experience in Grozny.

CONCLUSION

CF Transformation is ongoing to meet the non-linear, non-contiguous future battlespace. CSS organizations must review their current organization and doctrine to ensure they remain relevant in future operations. CFHS field ambulances are organizations that have limited relevance in current and future operations and should be realigned along modularized capabilities, as modular HSS organizations can provide surgical services, post-operative monitoring and ancillary equipment necessary to support casualties until they can be evacuated or returned to duty. Recent experiences of allied military medical organizations suggested that, while mobility was considered an important doctrinal planning factor, it was often sacrificed to ensure patient treatment, especially if the facilities were sited in defendable positions. Canadian support doctrine has acknowledged the relative immobility of much of the CSS assets expected to support a joint deployment by envisioning a joint camp in support of hub-and-spoke operations that is defendable. HSS support in this future joint camp is referred to as the Joint Health Support Unit, a modular facility with a structure and capabilities similar to the current Advanced Surgical Centres. Also, US experience suggested that their Combat Support Hospitals could be smaller facilities, making them closer in size and capability to an ASC. Further, UK medical units evacuated patients from Role 1 to Role 3 facilities, without stopping at Role 2 facilities in the chain of evacuation, because they had the ability to evacuate patients directly and quickly to the required treatment facility. This activity indicates that Role 2 facilities have limited utility in current and future operations, provided robust evacuation modules exist at Role 1 and Role 3 facilities to meet the evacuation demands. By replacing field ambulance structures with modules that include surgery modules, CFHS will be better positioned to meet the land component HSS requirements in asymmetric future operations.

However, before this debate can be resolved, further research is required to investigate the ongoing impact of the non-linear, non-continuous battlespace on the provision of HSS in future operations. Additionally, there is a requirement to conduct evidence-based studies on the efficacy of the medical skill sets required forward of definitive (trauma) surgery, so that limited HSS personnel and resources are appropriately employed to maximize patient survivability.

NOTES

1   Major G. Richardson, "Medical Support to the Army," briefing note to Chief of Staff Health Services, 6 March 1997.

2   David Salisbury and Allan English, "Prognosis 2020: A Military Medical Strategy for the Canadian Forces," *Canadian Military Journal* 4, no.2 (Summer 2003), 53. This essay is chapter 1 in this volume.

3   J.C. Taylor, "Whither the Field Ambulance? Role 2 Land Health Service Support in the 21st Century Battlespace," paper written for the Advanced Military Studies Course, CFC in 2002, 19. It appears as chapter 3 in this volume.

4   David Weger, "Blurring of the Lines: The Call for an Integrated Surgical Capability in Canadian Field Ambulances," paper written for the Advanced Military Studies Course, Canadian Forces College (2003). Weger's paper is Chapter 4 in this volume.

5   Canada, Department of National Defence (DND), *Canadian Forces Strategic Operating Concept, Draft 4.4* (Ottawa: Deputy Chief of the Defence Staff, 21 May 2004), para 14.

6   Ibid., para 87.

7   DND, *CF Joint Operating Concept 2012* (Draft) (Ottawa: DND, 24 July 2003), 12.

8   DND, "National Military Support Capability Concept of Operations," Annex C, Appendix 1-Joint Support Group Division of Responsibility Matrix, http://www.dcds.mil.ca/project/pmonmsc/default_e.asp, accessed 25 February 2005.

9   Discussions between the author and National Military Support Capability Working Group Chairpersons in Cornwall, ON, 25 February 2005.

10   Additional detailed explanations of each role's capability are in DND, *Health Services Support to Canadian Forces Operations* (Final Draft), GJ-005-410-/FO-000 (Ottawa: DND, 2005).

11   DND, Canadian Forces Medical Services, "Role 3 Health Services Support," file number DSP G2536, 3000-3-G2536-300 (CFMG), 1996, pp. D-13-2/5 and D-13-3/5.

12   Ibid., pp. D-13-3/5 – D-13-4/5.

13   Definitions of NATO HSS Roles are in *Health Services Support to Canadian Forces Operations (Final Draft)*.

14   Ibid., chapter 1, Section 108, para 1.c.

15   US Department of Defense (DoD), *Doctrine for Health Services Support in Joint Operations*, Joint Publication 4-02 (Washington, DC: DoD, April 1995), 26.

16   J.B. Peake. "Fielding a Medical Force to keep Soldiers Healthy" *Army* 53, no. 6 (June 2003), 19-20.

17   M.J. Roberts, et al., "The Experience of the Intensive Care Unit in a British Army Field Hospital during the 2003 Gulf Conflict," *Journal of the Royal Army Medical Corps* (2003), 284-290.

18   United Kingdom, Ministry of Defence (MoD), *Logistics*, Army Doctrine Publication Volume 3 (London: MoD, June 1996), para 0213.

19   UK, MoD, *Army Medical Service Core Doctrine Volume 4—Part 2 Hospital Care (Draft 2)* (London: MoD, March 2004), para 0116.

20   D.R. Porr, *To Be There, To Be Ready and To Save Lives* (Carlisle Barracks, PA: US Army War College Paper, 1993).

21   American College of Surgeons Committee on Trauma, *ATLS Student Course Manual*, 6th ed.

(Chicago: American College of Surgeons, 1997).

22   G. Cecchine, et al., *Army Medical Support to the Army After Next: Issues and Insights from the Medical Technology Workshop, 1999* (Santa Monica: RAND, 2000), 18.

23   Porr, *To Be There, To Be Ready and To Save Lives.*

24   S.F. Gouge, *Combat Health Support of the Transformation Force in 2015* (Carlisle Barracks, PA: US Army War College, 2001).

25   DND, *Health Services Support to Canadian Forces Operations (Final Draft)*, Chapter 2, Section 202, para 4.

26   Ibid., Chapter 2, Section 205, para 3.

27   Gouge, *Combat Health Support of the Transformation Force in 2015*, 21.

28   C.J. Hooton, "Medical Support for the FMF: Far in the Rear, Too Much Gear," *Marine Corps Gazette* 74, no. 4 (April 1990), 52.

29   A.M. Smith, "Care Delayed is Care Denied: Casualty Handling in Littoral Operations," *Naval War College Review* 52, no. 4 (Autumn 1999), 109-21; and James Harris, "My Two Wars," *The New York Times* (20 April 2003), 4, 9.

30   D.J. Cohen, "Lessons Learned After Action Report on Deployment to Iraq: Role of the Combat Support Hospital," *Outlook*, (Winter 2004); available from http://das.cs.amedd.army.mil/outlook1.htm; accessed 10 September 2005.

31   Peake, "Fielding a Medical Force to keep Soldiers Healthy," 19-20.

32   Discussion with Captain Neil Bagley, UK Medical Services, describing his observations as 1 (UK) Division's Operations Medical Planner in support of Operation TELIC in 2003.

33   Roberts, et al., "The Experience of the Intensive Care Unit in a British Army Field Hospital during the 2003 Gulf Conflict,"149.

34   Discussion with Captain Neil Bagley, UK Medical Services, describing his observations as 1 (UK) Division's Operations Medical Planner in support of Op TELIC in 2003.

35   M.J. Roberts, et al., "The Experience of the Intensive Care Unit in a British Army Field Hospital during the 2003 Gulf Conflict,"149.

36   Russell W. Glenn, et al., *Urban Combat Service Support Operations: The Shoulders of Atlas* (Santa Monica: RAND, 2003).

37   V.J. Goulding, Jr., "Back to the Future with Asymmetric Warfare," *Parameters* 30, no. 4 (Winter 2000-01), 21-30.

38   S.E. Johnson, et al., *New Challenges New Tools for Defense Decision Making* (Santa Monica: RAND, 2003), 40-45.

39   From a lecture on "Asymmetric Warfare" provided to AMSC 8, 28 September 2005 by Colonel K.D. Dickson, Joint Forces Staff College, National Defense University.

40   L.W. Grau and T.L. Thomas, "'Soft Log' and Concrete Canyons: Russian Urban Combat Logistics in Grozny," *Marine Corps Gazette* 83, no. 10 (October 1999), 67-75.

41   A.M. Smith, "The Influence of Medicine on Strategy," *Naval War College Review* 41, no.2 (Spring 1988), 30.

42   Cecchine, et al., *Army Medical Support to the Army After Next*, 22.

43   Ibid., 23.

44   Ibid., 22.

45   Ibid., 23-4.

46   Ibid., 21.

47   Smith, "The Influence of Medicine on Strategy," 30.

48   M.J. Roberts, et al., "The Experience of the Intensive Care Unit in a British Army Field Hospital during the 2003 Gulf Conflict,"149.

CHAPTER 6

DENTAL HEALTH SERVICES SUPPORT TO DEPLOYED CANADIAN FORCES OPERATIONS IN 2020

Major Stephen Molyneaux

INTRODUCTION

The history of dental support to Canadian soldiers is as long as the nation's history of operating abroad. In 1902, two civilian dentists accompanied the Canadian expeditionary force to South Africa during the Boer War and Canada's first military medical organization, the Army Medical Corps, established in 1904, had a contingent of militia dental officers. Uniformed dental service in the regular force began in the First World War with the formation of the Royal Canadian Dental Corps in 1915, and continued during the Second World War and the Korean War in dental clinics mounted on vehicles. These mobile facilities were a technological marvel at the time, and were not dissimilar in concept to those in service today. As Canada shifted from warfighting to operations other than war following the Korean conflict, the renamed Canadian Forces Dental Services (CFDS) kept pace. Dental personnel have served in all of Canada's major overseas peace support missions, including the current mission to Afghanistan. Through variations in size and structure, the CFDS has been an integral part of the health service support (HSS) provided to Canada's deployed operations.

Along with most other capabilities of the Canadian Forces (CF), the operational capabilities of the CFDS face the need for major changes due to the new international security environment and advances in military technology. In 1999, the Chief of the Defence Staff released *Shaping the Future of the Canadian Forces: A Strategy for 2020 (Strategy 2020)*, a strategic vision for the CF in the 21st century. Intended to "guide our planning, force structure and procurement decisions, as well as our investments in personnel, education and training," *Strategy 2020* laid out a series of strategic objectives for the CF.[1] This paper will examine these objectives as they pertain to operational dentistry in the year 2020, and make a number of recommendations for changes to better meet these objectives. It will argue that the main change needed for dental HSS to support global operations in 2020 is the adoption of a single capability module, meaning a common "building block" for the task of providing clinical dental treatment to a deployed force, either independently or as part of a group of modules.[2] This capability module would include both trained personnel and their equipment, and must be readily deployable, modern, and interoperable with our allies. The module must be simple in concept and sophisticated in capability. To achieve these capabilities, changes in equipment, organization and doctrine will be required.

This chapter begins by examining current dental HSS capabilities. It then discusses dental HSS considerations in the future operating environment. Finally, the chapter discusses what changes in equipment, organization and doctrine will be required for dental HSS to meet the *Strategy 2020* objectives of globally deployable, modernize, and interoperable as they relate to the HSS principles of proximity, flexibility, and mobility, and also to the operational principle of war of simplicity.[3]

As HSS to the land force is considered to be the most complex HSS activity due to the mobility and dispersion of land forces, this chapter will focus on land operations, although the conclusions could be applied to the maritime and air components.[4] Regarding the CFDS, this chapter will consider only dental HSS to deployed operations and no other aspects of that organization.

STRATEGIC GUIDANCE

Strategy 2020 laid out the following vision for the CF over the next two decades:

> The Defence Team will generate, employ and sustain high-quality, combat-capable, interoperable and rapidly deployable task-tailored forces. We will exploit leading-edge doctrine and technologies to accomplish our domestic and international roles in the battlespace of the 21st century and be recognized, both at home and abroad, as an innovative, relevant knowledge-based institution. With transformational leadership and coherent management, we will build upon our proud heritage in pursuit of clear strategic objectives.[5]

These strategic objectives, the "essence of *Strategy 2020*," are intended to guide defence planning over the next two decades and give *Strategy 2020* a "practical effect." [6] The objectives are: innovative path, decisive leaders, modernize, globally deployable, interoperable, career of choice, strategic partnerships, and resource stewardship. [7] Although all of these objectives have some applicability to any element of the CF, the three strategic objectives of globally deployable, modernize, and interoperable have the most relevance for dental HSS.

The Army built on the vision for the CF laid out in *Strategy 2020* and implemented a strategy for the land force in its document *Advancing with Purpose: The Army Strategy*, released in 2002. The document described the Army of Today, from the present to five years from now, the Army of Tomorrow, 5 to 10 years from the present, and the Future Army, beyond 10 years. The Army in 2020 will therefore be the Future Army, but decisions affecting any capabilities of this force will be taken during the period embracing the Armies of Today and Tomorrow. Of particular note to dental HSS is the recognition that sustainability, including the long-term physical health of personnel, will be a decisive point for the Army. An objective with a 10-year target for realization is the transformation of the Army into a "medium weight, information-age" force. [8] This transformation will influence any dental HSS capabilities operating with the land force in 2020.

CURRENT DENTAL HSS CAPABILITIES

Health care is recognized by *Strategy 2020* as an issue that will continue to be a high priority for Canadians and thus for the CF. [9] The CF is morally and legally obliged to provide health care to its personnel, whether in garrison or deployed. The list of medical and dental treatments that the CF has committed to provide to its members is extensive and similar to civilian standards. [10]

The CFDS and the Canadian Forces Medical Services are branches of the Canadian Forces Health Services (CFHS). In a land setting, the role of both medical and dental HSS is to conserve personnel strength for commanders. [11] In garrison and in the field, dental capabilities in Canada belong to the Canadian Forces Health Services Group (CF H Svcs Gp). Overseas dental assets belong to the Task Force Commander through some form of deployed composite HSS unit, with CF H Svcs Gp maintaining professional/technical control.

CFHS is currently undergoing major reforms and reorganization to correct past difficulties with medical care provided to the CF.[12] These initiatives are discussed in detail in Chapters 1 and 8 of this book. Future medical and dental HSS to deployed operations will be affected by the proposed changes from the Standing Committee on Operational Medicine Review, including the identification of operational clinical capabilities as separately deployable modules.[13] These changes represent a shift from the current emphasis on clinical capabilities at the unit level, or those organized on an ad hoc basis for particular deployments.

The principal dental HSS equipment for field use at present is the Mobile Dental Clinic (MDC), which is a dental clinic in a metal shelter carried on a "Medium Logistic Vehicle Wheeled." These MDCs are distributed mainly to CF H Svcs Gp's three field ambulances, and its single field hospital and dental training institution. Dental personnel in these field units are organized into platoons, each with four treatment sections consisting of a dental officer and two dental technicians. The CF has enough MDCs to equip approximately 30 treatment sections, roughly half of which are currently in operational units. The other half of these treatment sections would be drawn from garrison personnel in support of contingency operations plans. Although it possesses many capabilities, the present MDC was designed in the 1970s and entered service in the early 1980s. As such, it is legacy equipment for the CF.

Medical and dental HSS is currently categorized into various roles defined by function and location,[14] and CFHS definitions of HSS roles are compliant with NATO definitions.[15] Role 1 dental care is very basic emergency treatment provided at or near the patient's initial location, but not necessarily by dental personnel. Role 2 dental care is sustaining care provided by dental personnel, including emergency care and simple non-emergency dental treatment. This level of care is normally provided at the field ambulance. Role 3 dental care is maintaining care, more comprehensive treatment provided at the field hospital level, involving dental specialists and an integral surgical capability. Role 4 is rehabilitative care provided out of theatre, including the most complex dental treatments. Medical roles are similar, with Roles 1 to 3 being respectively -

emergency care, stabilization, and initial surgery. On current peace support missions, a single deployed dental treatment section with an MDC provides Role 1 and 2 levels of care. This ability of a single section to operate across multiple HSS roles, a current strength of dental HSS, must be maintained and strengthened in the future dental capability module.

DENTAL HSS CONSIDERATIONS IN THE FUTURE OPERATING ENVIRONMENT

It is likely that, in the future, HSS will be required for a wide variety of overseas operations, and health care planning scenarios requiring dental support range from disaster relief to international humanitarian missions to warfighting in collective defence.[16] Future dental HSS capabilities must, therefore, be flexible and robust enough to operate in any of these scenarios.

Warfighting will likely involve smaller, more potent forces, with sophisticated command and control that will allow the force to be widely dispersed in the theatre of operations.[17] These conflicts will occur quickly, with less build up of forces and shorter durations.[18] The Canadian Army has adopted manoeuvre warfare as its concept for warfighting,[19] and the challenge for HSS assets in such future warfighting operations will be to have sufficient mobility and agility to keep up with the supported forces, rather than the capacity and endurance to treat large numbers of patients.

For operations other than war, especially humanitarian relief to impoverished areas of the world, the challenge will be reversed and the capacity to treat large numbers of patients will be required.[20] Canadian military dental assets have yet to be deployed on a mission solely to provide care to a civilian population, but it cannot be assumed that they will never be deployed to a humanitarian crisis for such a reason, especially considering that civilian substitutes for this specialized capability are rare. The Disaster Assistance Response Team deployment to Sri Lanka in early 2005 may be the forerunner of many such HSS humanitarian missions.

The physical environment in recent dental HSS deployments has included such varied environments as the hot and dusty climate of Afghanistan and the cold conditions of the Ontario/Quebec ice storm of 1998. Future deployments will see more of the same, and could also see land deployments to humid tropical forests of Sub-Saharan Africa and the extreme cold of Canada's far north; therefore, dental HSS capabilities must be able to operate in all of these environments.[21] This requirement has been and will continue to be a challenge for some sensitive dental equipment.

For warfighting and peace support operations, the deployed patient population will be members of the CF. The initial warfighting force will likely be smaller, with highly skilled personnel who arrive in theatre and begin their mission quickly. While the loss of a single member of this force due to health issues could have grave consequences,[22] traditionally CF dental HSS has been provided only for land deployments of battle group size and greater, and it may not be efficient to deploy CF dental HSS assets in support of smaller future warfighting forces.

One way of addressing this situation would be to raise the dental fitness level for those CF members with a high likelihood of deploying in small groups, such as special operations forces. The CFDS uses NATO classification standards for dental fitness, with Class 1 dental fitness meaning that the patient has no requirement for any type of dental treatment at all, Class 2 dental fitness meaning a need for emergency dental treatment is not anticipated within 12 months,[23] and Class 3 and Class 4 patients have oral health conditions rendering them unfit for deployment. The great majority of CF members, being in Class 2 with a lesser number in Class 1, are thus considered fit for deployment. However, for those highly deployable and irreplaceable warfighters described above, a Class 1 dental fitness may be required at all times. This is a meticulous standard and would be difficult to implement due to treatment time requirements, but reflects the high state of overall health that personnel may require when operating without ready access to traditional medical and dental HSS. Currently, this patient group is less likely to be at Class 1 dental fitness than some other groups due to competing time demands which make group members less available for dental treatment. The US Army has set a goal of shifting "the majority of soldiers from Class 2 to Class 1" for its Army After Next, a very ambitious goal for that force.[24]

Due to their need for extensive human interactions, future peace support missions will not see the same reduction in numbers or duration as warfighting missions have over time. Similarly, future periods of intense conflict with smaller forces may be followed by larger stabilization forces deployed for a longer period.[25] The CF will continue engaging in these larger types of missions, so robust dental HSS capabilities will need to be maintained. The most effective means of preserving personnel strength for commanders will remain the ability to prevent dental casualties, and to treat those casualties that do arise far forward and allow for a quick return to duty, the two HSS principles of mobility and proximity.[26] Preventative care provided in garrison and by deployed dental HSS assets will remain the services that most effectively support commanders for future CF land operations.[27] For humanitarian missions to civilian populations, a capacity to treat large numbers of patients with very high dental treatment needs will be required.

Considerations for future dental HSS roles and the characteristics of the dental capability module for deployed operations is closely tied to the ongoing debate on whether the roles for HSS as currently defined will have much relevance for future operations, especially warfighting opera-tions. Some have argued that the traditional Role 2 of stabilization will no longer be necessary as "brilliant medics," exceptionally well-trained and with advanced technology, will stabilize casualties at Role 1, allowing for evacuation directly to what are now the facilities of initial surgery and hospitalization at Role 3.[28] Others have argued that Role 2 HSS units with enhanced evacuation and surgical capability will remain relevant in the 21st century.[29] In the CF, field ambulances, in which a large portion of current dental HSS assets is traditionally located, provide Role 2 care. The long-term fate of the field ambulance is thus of great interest to dental HSS planners.

For dental HSS, the answer to the question of roles will be to structure itself around a single dental capability module comprised of one new MDC staffed by one dental treatment section. This module must be able to function as the sole dental capability in theatre for Roles 1 through 3, and thus must be equipped for all but the most complex dental treatments. If more than one module is required, additional modules can be deployed and "task tailored" for the specific operation.[30] The proper location of each module will be dictated by the need to treat and quickly return to duty as many patients as possible, and may be either with a larger HSS unit or independent of the same. This flexibility is a principle of HSS, and can be employed more readily for dental HSS because of its more limited range of functions as compared to medical HSS. This limited range of functions is reflected in the effect of the debate of HSS roles on dental HSS in the CF. Even though the definitions of roles are tending to become more complex in developing CF HSS doctrine, with Roles 1 and 2 gaining "enhanced" sub-categories,[31] and though these definitions may remain relevant for medical HSS, units structured to provide defined Roles are not critical for current dental HSS and will be less important in the future. Larger HSS units such as the field ambulance and field hospital, because they are unlikely to deploy as a single unit in the future, should then function as garrison holding units for the MDCs and treatment sections of each dental HSS capability module, rather than as clinically deployable entities themselves.   The focus of attention should be on making each module as independent and as clinically comprehensive as possible, and the capability module can be seen as an attempt to provide standardization and order to the ad hoc HSS clinical structures currently reactively provided by units for each deployment.

The number of dental capability modules required in 2020 will depend on the size of the CF. The current fleet of approximately 30 MDCs were acquired for a 1970s era CF, which had a strength of about 80,000 personnel, and was larger than the force today, which currently stands at about 60,000 personnel. If the CF returns to a strength of 80,000 personnel, a modestly decreased fleet of 25 MDCs would be sufficient to support the recent CF operations tempo, as well as training requirements and contingency operations plans. Historically, however, dental treatment requirements of a deployed force have not varied with the type of operation, and instead the number of patients in need of dental treatment has been a function of the size of the supported force and its baseline oral health.[32] This relation is not likely to change in 2020, and one dental module staffed by a dental officer and two dental technicians will continue to be sufficient to meet the treatment needs of a battle group sized deployment. Therefore, garrison treatment requirements rather than operational requirements will be the determining factor for the personnel strength of the CFDS needed to serve the future force.

The roles of uniformed HSS personnel have been debated in recent literature. Specifically, the role traditionally filled by deployed medical officers may be filled by other medical personnel operating with advanced medical technology. Furthermore, in the CF, the traditional role of physicians is changing regardless of technology due to the chronic shortage of medical officers.[33] However, the specific technical knowledge and very particular psychomotor skills required to deliver dental treatment, and the fact that dental problems are usually non-life threatening and thus allow time for patient transport prior to treatment, make it unlikely that dental officers will need to be replaced in the same way. These facts suggest that current staffing levels for dental officers and technicians are appropriate.

The question of whether the CFDS could be disbanded and dental care outsourced to civilian providers was examined in the 1990s. It was determined then that the chief reason for maintaining a uniformed dental service was the fact that it would be very difficult, if not impossible, to provide dental care in a theatre of operations with civilian providers. Given this fact, the CFDS is an organization that has given the highest priority to providing personnel for deployed operations, and will certainly continue to do so in the future.

How dental HSS capabilities could be made more effective to meet the challenges of the future operating environment will be examined next using relevant criteria from *Strategy 2020*.

STRATEGY 2020 OBJECTIVE: GLOBALLY DEPLOYABLE

Based on the strategic objective of globally deployable, *Strategy 2020* seeks to "enhance the combat preparedness, global deployability and sustainability of our maritime, land and air forces." Two specific targets are a vanguard and main contingency force "fully deployable to an offshore theatre of operations within 21 and 90 days respectively" and to "enhance our strategic airlift and sealift capability."[34] Implications for dental HSS from this emphasis of deployability are to be found in both the future patient population and future dental capabilities.

Both the CF and the US Army have recognized that dental HSS should be deployable as modules.[35] Flexibility and simplicity will be the key concepts for the equipping of the CF dental capability module in 2020; therefore, the module should be deployable in a variety of modes. When medium lift is available, both the metal shelter containing the treatment facility and its prime mover vehicle would be transported to the theatre. When only light lift is available or mobility is not critical, as in a static peace support mission, the shelter would be transported without its prime mover. In either case, the supporting equipment required for dental treatment, such as the power generator and air compressor, would be fixed to the shelter but detachable. No auxiliary trailer would be required to operate the clinic. This supporting equipment must be as light and quiet as possible for deployability and tactical utility in the field. Current MDCs require a noisy and outdated generator on a separate trailer.

When only very minimal transport is available, the same dental equipment used inside the metal shelter would be shipped into theatre without the shelter, accompanied by the same supporting equipment detached from the shelter. In this way, the same equipment could be employed in a variety of modes as determined by the needs of the mission and available transport. This change would be an improvement over the current situation, in which different equipment is used for air transportation of a lighter equipment set, vice sea transportation of the MDC. As this air transportable equipment is different, it presents separate training requirements, which are difficult to fulfill due to the limited number of sets available.

The shelter employed should be a standard sized shipping container to facilitate transport by sea, air, and road. A project to replace the Army's medium truck fleet, and possibly its existing specialized shelters, is being developed, and the preliminary submission for a new dental shelter contains many of the features suggested above.[36]

In a warfighting mission, HSS mobility will be critical to keep up with the highly mobile and dispersed supported force, and thus a prime mover for the MDC would be required. Excellent communications equipment for situational awareness and the ability to deploy quickly to future conflicts will be other essentials for warfighting HSS.[37] Dental modules will also need to be self-contained for independent operation, as future commanders may consider deployed dental capability modules without these characteristics as more of a hindrance than an asset. Even in a static operation other than war in which the prime mover is not deployed, good communications, rapid deployability, and independent operation will be requirements of dental HSS modules in 2020. At present, the communication ability of the MDC fleet is poor to non-existent, leaving the dental section very dependent on other elements for situational awareness. The dental sections staffing these modules naturally will need to be well trained and qualified to perform their dental functions. The recent case of US Army combat service support personnel being captured during the invasion of Iraq when their convoy took a wrong turn demonstrates that support personnel will also need to be well trained in military skills in the non-contiguous battlespace environment of future operations. For HSS personnel, this need extends to their Geneva Convention duty to defend their patients as well as themselves.[38]

STRATEGY 2020 OBJECTIVE: MODERNIZE

The *Strategy 2020* objective of modernize is to:

> Field a viable and affordable force structure trained and equipped to generate advanced combat capabilities that target leading edge doctrine and technologies relevant to the battlespace of the 21st century.[39]

As is the case for other capabilities throughout the CF, the dental capability module in 2020 will employ advanced technologies. In the case of HSS, advanced technologies will be necessary to keep up with evolving civilian standards of care. However, over reliance on technology in developing future HSS capabilities ought to be avoided since some future health technologies may turn out to be too expensive or not viable for military applications.[40] For dental HSS, this caveat means that well qualified personnel will remain the core of the dental capability module rather than the equipment.

Nevertheless, the current fleet of MDCs is three decades old in design, and in need of replacement. The standard of care expected from deployed CF HSS for future missions will be equivalent to the standard of care accessible to most Canadians within one or two hours.[41] For dental HSS, this requirement means that deployable dental capability modules must keep up with the technology of a modern civilian dental office. The current MDC is falling behind in this regard. Of particular interest will be information management and telecommunications, two areas noted as important for research and development in *Strategy 2020*.[42] For dental HSS, the deployed module must have access to computerized dental records to remain both up to date technologically and able to comply with legislative requirements for health record keeping.[43] The patient's same full digital record would then be available across the continuum of in-garrison and deployed dental HSS. At present, the deployed team generates a temporary paper dental record and does not have access to the full paper dental record. A digital radiography capability will also be an important means of exchanging information between deployed dental teams and specialists at home, and will have lighter equipment requirements than traditional film radiography.[44]

Another area of interest related to modernization will be future standards for infection control and environmental protection. The current MDC was designed when these factors were of lesser concern than they are today. Since high infection risk treatment will be performed in the replacement MDC, the shelter must have surfaces that are easily disinfected to modern infection control standards.[45] From an environmental protection perspective, the wastewater generated by dental treatment must be safely stored and disposed of when proper facilities are available to the deployed module. As is becoming the standard in the civilian sector, mercury will also need to be separated from this wastewater.[46]

In addition to its equipment, training for the personnel of the dental section in 2020 will have to reflect modern practices, both military and civilian. One necessary step will be to update the tactical doctrine concerning the future dental HSS module. Current doctrine described in the 1992 publication *Dental Services in Battle* is out of date.[47] It should be updated after the operational HSS doctrine currently being promulgated is ratified.[48] The updated doctrine should have useful and up to date information on dental subjects such as infection control and military subjects such as the future battlespace. It should also emphasize the dental capability module as the fundamental building block for dental HSS.

STRATEGY 2020 OBJECTIVE: INTEROPERABLE

To enhance interoperability, *Strategy 2020* seeks to:

> Strengthen our military to military relationships with our principal allies ensuring interoperable forces, doctrine, and C4I (command, control, communications, computers, and intelligence).[49]

Interoperability with the armed forces of our principal ally, the United States, is recognized as being of pre-eminent importance in Canadian doctrine.[50] For dental HSS in 2020 this objective means having similar capabilities as the three US Dental Corps.

Currently, dental HSS interoperability with US forces is fair. Some equipment is used in common between the CFDS and its American counterparts in their three services, and the dental treatment capabilities of deployed sections are essentially the same. Furthermore, Canadian dental officers do most of their post-graduate training, in particular for Advanced General Dentistry, which is a major speciality occupation for both forces, at US Army dental training facilities.[51]

However, there are some developments concerning our interoperability with the United States that could prove to be a difficulty in 2020. US Armed Forces dental officers have a paramedical role as triage officers in mass casualty situations that could arise during any warfighting or unstable peace support mission.[52] Current CF HSS doctrine recognizes a paramedical role for dental officers, but the specific role of triage officer in mass casualty situations is at risk of being lost.[53] This discrepancy may limit the future ability of Canadian dental officers to operate within American HSS facilities.

Canada does meet, and should be able to continue to meet, the specific capabilities specified for NATO nations in deployable Role 1 to 3 dental care.[54] However, as treatment roles become increasingly blurred, the treatment requirements will remain, and CF dental HSS modules must continue to fill them. Interoperability with nations other than the United States could be problematic because the standard of dental care in some parts of the world is in many ways dissimilar to that of the US and

Canada. The practical implication of this fact for 2020 will be that if Canada is involved in a combined mission with nations for which this lower standard is a concern, then the CF will be obliged to ensure that its personnel receive care of an acceptable standard. This situation will be more likely to arise in the future as more countries join NATO.

CONCLUSION

The CFDS must meet the strategic objectives laid out in *Strategy 2020* of globally deployable, modernize, and interoperable. The CFDS should, therefore, develop a new dental capability module, consisting of one dental treatment section and associated replacement MDC, as the standardized and sophisticated building block on which to structure dental HSS to overseas missions. The dental capability module should be able to accomplish all tasks for dental Roles 1 through 3, and the MDC for the 2020 dental capability module should be flexible enough to deploy in a variety of modes as the mission demands and available transport allows. For simplicity, the same dental and support equipment should be used in all of these modes. Moreover, deployed dental capability modules must have excellent communications ability and be able to operate independently.

To replace the aging MDC fleet, the new dental shelter and its associated equipment should be modern, including advanced computer technology for patient records. The future dental module must meet 2020 civilian standards in infection control and environmental protection. Further, dental tactical doctrine should be updated to reflect the emphasis on the dental capability module, and dental personnel must be well trained as both clinical and military professionals.

The CFDS is capable now of limited interoperability with the armed forces of the United States. This capability should be enhanced. Likewise, while CF dental HSS meets the standards of our NATO allies, we must also continue to ensure that Canadian dental standards of care are available to CF personnel on all combined deployments. The CF should be prepared to be the lead nation for dental support when the Canadian standard of dental care is not readily available from contributing coalition partners.

Seeing these recommendations fully realized would not be a simple task. Dental HSS benefits from being part of a larger HSS organization through access to necessary but non-integral capabilities. At the same time, the need for conformity within this HSS organization may inhibit the application of solutions specifically suited for dental HSS. Of course, fiscal realities also remain a limiting factor. The CFDS has a proud history of support to Canada's overseas military deployments and to continue to fulfill this role dental HSS to overseas missions must meet the vision and strategic objectives of *Strategy 2020*.

NOTES

1   Canada, Department of National Defence (DND), *Shaping the Future of the Canadian Forces: A Strategy for 2020* (Ottawa: DND, 1999), 1.

2   DND, Director General Health Services, *Standing Committee on Operational Medicine Review: Phase One Final Report* (henceforth *SCOMR 1*) (Ottawa: CFHS, 2001), 77.

3   DND, *Health Services Support to Canadian Forces Operations (Ratification Draft)*, B-GJ-005-410/FP-000 (Ottawa: DND, 2004), p. 1-5; and Canadian Forces College, "Contemporary Principles of War," Command and Staff Course 31 Activity Package C/JC/WTH 304/SM-1.

4   DND, *Canadian Forces Medical Group - Concept of Operations*, C/AS/JCP/J/LCP/DOC/L-7 (Ottawa: DND, 1997), 3.

5   DND, *Shaping the Future of the Canadian Forces: A Strategy for 2020*, 8.

6   Ibid., 9.

7   Ibid., 10-12.

8   Ibid., 3, 8, 16, 20.

9   Ibid., 5.

10   DND, Director General Health Services, "Spectrum of Care," http://www.forces.gc.ca/health/services/engraph/spectrum_of_care_home_e.asp; accessed 4 January 2005.

11   DND, *Health Service Support*, B-GL-343-001/FP-00 (Ottawa: DND, 2001), 2,127.

12   D.A. Salisbury, "Prescription 2020: Considerations for a Military Medical Strategy for the Canadian Forces," paper written for National Security Studies Course (NSSC) 4 (Toronto: Canadian Forces College, October 2002), 3.

13   DND, *SCOMR 1*, 1-2, 77.

14   DND, *Health Services Support to Canadian Forces Operations (Ratification Draft)*, p. 1-8.

15   North Atlantic Treaty Organization (NATO), *Allied Joint Medical Support Doctrine*, AJP-4.10 (henceforth *AJP-4.10*) (Brussels: NATO Standardization Agency, 2002), 16-18.

16   DND, *SCOMR 1*, Annex K, 22-3.

17   Scott Beaty, "The Revolution in Military Medical Affairs," *Parameters* 27 no. 4 (Winter 1997), 5.

18   S.F. Gouge, *Combat Health Support of the Transformation Force in 2015*, (Carlisle Barracks, PA: US Army War College, 2001), 21.

19   DND, *Health Service Support*, 4.

20   Beaty, "The Revolution in Military Medical Affairs," 9.

21   DND, *Health Service Support*, 117.

22   Salisbury, "Prescription 2020," 10.

23   NATO, Military Agency for Standardization (MAS), *Dental Fitness Standards for Military Personnel and a Dental Fitness Classification System*, STANAG 2466, edition 1 (Brussels: MAS, 1999), pp. A-1, B-1.

24   Conrad F. Bodai, *Dental Support for the Army After Next* (Carlisle Barracks, PA: US Army War College Paper, 1998), 19.

25   Ibid., 9.

26   DND, *Health Services Support to Canadian Forces Operations (Ratification Draft)*, p. 1-5.

27   DND, *SCOMR 1*, 36.

28   Beaty, "The Revolution in Military Medical Affairs," 6.

29   J.C. Taylor, "Whither the Field Ambulance? Role 2 Land Health Service Support in the 21st Century Battlespace," 19-20, paper written for the Advanced Military Studies Course, CFC in 2002. It appears as chapter 3 in this volume.

30   DND, *Shaping the Future of the Canadian Forces: A Strategy for 2020*, 8.

31   DND, *Health Services Support to Canadian Forces Operations (Ratification Draft)*, pp. 6-5 to 6-8.

32   US Army, *Dental Service Support in a Theater of Operations*, Field Manual 4-02.19 (Washington: Department of the Army, 2001), 3-13, http://atiam.train.army.mil/portal/atia/adlsc/view/public/297025-1/fm/4-02.19/fm4-02.19.htm; accessed 12 December 2004.

33   Salisbury, "Prescription 2020," 19.

34   DND, *Shaping the Future of the Canadian Forces: A Strategy for 2020*, 11.

35   For the CF see DND, *SCOMR 1*, Annex K, 16; and for the US Army see *Dental Service Support in a Theater of Operations*, 2-5.

36   Personal communication, Deputy Chief of Staff Dental Services 3-2 and author, December 2004.

37   Gouge, *Combat Health Support of the Transformation Force in 2015*, 22, 25.

38   DND, Office of the Judge Advocate General, "Geneva Convention (I) for the Amelioration of the Condition of the Wounded and Sick in Armed Forces in the Field - 1949," in Directorate of Law Training (DLT), ed., *Collection of Documents on the Law of Armed Conflict* (Ottawa: DLT, 2004), 71.

39   DND, *Shaping the Future of the Canadian Forces: A Strategy for 2020*, 10.

40   G. Cecchine, et al., *Army Medical Strategy: Issues for the Future*, report Prepared for the US Army Medical Department (Santa Monica: RAND Arroyo Center, 2001), 32, 38, http://handle.dtic.mil/100.2/ADA400828; accessed 12 December 2004.

41   DND, *SCOMR 1*, 2.

42   DND, *Shaping the Future of the Canadian Forces: A Strategy for 2020*, 10.

43   Royal College of Dental Surgeons of Ontario (RCDSO), *Dental Recordkeeping* (Toronto: RCDSO, 2002), 2.

44   Bodai, *Dental Support for the Army After Next*, 11.

45   Royal College of Dental Surgeons of Ontario, *Infection Control in the Dental Office* (Toronto: RCDSO, 2002), 3, 6.

46   Albert O. Adegbembo and Philip A. Watson, "Estimated Quantity of Mercury in Amalgam Waste Water Residue Released by Dentists into the Sewerage System in Ontario Canada," *Journal of the Canadian Dental Association* 70 no. 11 (December 2004), 759.

47   DND, *Dental Services in Battle*, B-GL-312-012/FP-001 (Ottawa: DND, 1992), pp. 1-4-1, 2-1-1, 2-2-1.

48   DND, *Health Services Support to Canadian Forces Operations (Ratification Draft)*, ix.

49   DND, *Shaping the Future of the Canadian Forces: A Strategy for 2020*, 11.

50   Ibid., 9.

51   Russell J. Czerw, *Changes in the Army Dental Corps: Supporting Transformation* (Carlisle Barracks, PA: US Army War College Paper, 2002), 16.

52   US Department of Defense (DoD), *Doctrine for Health Services Support in Joint Operations,* Joint Publication 4-02 (Washington, DC: DoD, 2001), p. III-8.

53   DND, *SCOMR 1*, 17.

54   NATO, MAS, *Tasks for the Appropriate Staffing and Training of Dental Officers and Ancillary Personnel for Wartime Operations and Operational Deployments*, STANAG 2465, edition 1 (Brussels: MAS, 1999), iii.

CHAPTER 7

FIGHTING FIT: SUSTAINING THE FORCE BY FIXING AFLOAT HEALTH SERVICE SUPPORT ON THE JOINT SUPPORT SHIP

Commander Rebecca Patterson

Regardless of the location of medical support facilities in any littoral strategy, however, a historical perspective remains: the sick
and injured are perishable cargo and the ordinary rules of logistics cannot be applied to them.[1]

Captain Arthur Smith, Medical Corps, US Naval Reserve (retired)

INTRODUCTION

Detailed planning is underway for the Canadian Navy's Joint Support Ship
(JSS), a replacement for the aging Preserver Class Auxiliary Oil
Replenishment (AOR) vessels. The JSS will be a multipurpose ship that
will provide surge sealift, underway replenishment, and support to forces
ashore. It will include a level of medical coverage that exceeds anything
currently provided by the Canadian Navy.[2] With the announcement in
June 2006 of $2.9 billion for the JSS project, the first of three vessels is
scheduled for completion in 2012.[3] Once deployed, the JSS is expected to
provide a comprehensive joint capability to a Canadian Forces Task
Group, and has the potential to serve as a leader in the drive towards
establishing Canadian Forces (CF) joint operational capability.[4] Paul
Mitchell underscored the potential significance of the JSS when he stated,
"the JSS may mark the transition of the Navy…to a more land-support-
oriented mission. It also may drag the entire Canadian Forces kicking
and screaming into being a fully fledged joint institution." With the existing AORs rapidly reaching the end of their life cycle, the JSS project, as
the vanguard of future CF jointness, is facing considerable pressure to
meet the timelines for the production of the first ship.[5]

The JSS Medical Capability Working Group identified an operational requirement for an enhanced surgical and hospital capability on the JSS from what is currently available on the existing AORs. A limited Role 3 capability,[6] in the form of an integral JSS Afloat Advanced Surgical Centre (AASC)[7] has been identified to meet the potential force planning scenarios of the future. This capability can be increased to accommodate a scalable, modularized, joint Enhanced Afloat Advanced Surgical Centre (EAASC)[8] should the operational requirement exist. However, the delivery of sea-based joint limited Role 3 health service support (HSS) of this scalability and capability is a new and exciting venture for both the Navy and the CF.[9]

The challenge to effectively utilize this resource- and space-intensive capability will be directly impacted by the multipurpose function of the JSS. Multiple, divergent taskings required from a single JSS will result in competing and sometimes incompatible demands being placed on the platform. This will be particularly true if a role 3 HSS capability has been committed to a Joint Task Force (JTF) operation. The JTF Commander must therefore exercise extreme caution when assigning other tasks to the JSS to prevent the undermining of the theatre HSS, as the JSS-based Role 3 capability will likely be the only CF capability of this type in the Area of Operations (AO).[10] Resolving the debate of how and when the sea-based Role 3 HSS capability is to be employed will be essential to prevent the afloat medical facility from becoming, in Mitchell's words, a "white elephant" that consumes limited financial and human resources while offering little added value.[11]

Enhanced joint sea-based medical capability will be an efficient use of scarce HSS resources if HSS planners and JTF Commanders adhere to the concepts of operational HSS planning and delivery and commit, prior to construction, to utilizing the capability effectively. This chapter will demonstrate that adherence to these concepts has the potential to impact the multipurpose function of the JSS by limiting its mobility, and therefore, its ability to carry out other activities for the Naval Task Group. These limitations must be acceptable to the JTF Commander prior to leaving the homeport in order to ensure that joint, sea-based Role 3 HSS is an operational capability rather than an operational liability to the JTF Commander.

Operational commanders forecast battle casualty rates and exercise responsibility for the health and welfare of the force as part of Force Health Protection, and they exercise this responsibility through the HSS supporting elements. The primary objective of force health protection is to conserve the fighting strength of the force through the spectrum of health services - from preventive health measures to delivery of advanced medical and surgical care for the sick and wounded.[12] During expeditionary operations, health service support, with few exceptions, is provided by CF Health Services personnel and equipment because relying on other nations to provide operational HSS is, in general, neither reliable nor morally acceptable for the CF.[13] Every effort is made to provide CF-based health care, and the JSS has the potential to be a more efficient platform to deliver this care when compared to the existing land-based Advanced Surgical Centres (ASC) or the minimal capabilities existing on the current AORs.

In order to provide context for the discussion, this chapter will provide an overview of the current status and issues surrounding the JSS project and briefly address the future of modern littoral warfare. This chapter will not address either the issues concerning the utility of other JSS capabilities or the integral sick bay capabilities of the JSS, rather it will focus exclusively on the issues surrounding sea-based, joint Role 3 HSS capabilities as the size and extent of this capability is a new venture for the CF. The chapter begins with a background discussion of factors related to the threats, risks and benefits of situating Role 3 HSS on a sea-based platform that must be considered by JTF Commander prior to deploying the JSS on a medical mission. This will include a discussion on the issues surrounding the employment of a large medical capability on a non-Geneva Convention-protected platform, as the JSS will not be designated as a hospital ship. A brief discussion about the future of sea-based HSS will then be provided, followed by a review of the concepts of HSS planning that, if properly adhered to, will impact the multipurpose function of the JSS. These critical concepts include timely access to health care, the "Golden Hour" for surgical intervention, and evacuation of casualties to and from the JSS platform. Finally, risk mitigation strategies will be briefly discussed, with the aim of suggesting ways in which to support the multipurpose function of the JSS without unduly placing casualties at risk of increased mortality or morbidity. The context of this chapter is based on the worst case peace support operational scenario where land and sea-based threats place the JSS at risk, as this will be the situation when multi-tasking capabilities will be critical to the CF. This context will also serve to illustrate the identification of the conditions that must exist in order to make sea-based Role 3 HSS a force enabling capability, rather than liability.

THE JSS CONTEXT

Knowledge of the JSS outside of the Canadian Navy is limited. An understanding of the issues surrounding the JSS concept and employment will, therefore, provide context for the operational requirement for sea-based Role 3 HSS. The Navy has envisioned the JSS as a multipurpose, combat capable ship that can provide strategic sealift, underway replenishment, and a command and control capability for a variety of joint and combined operational scenarios.[14]   The JSS will be capable of contributing to operational requirements for the full spectrum of domestic, continental and international planning scenarios, including Arctic operations, as a result of first year ice breaking capability. Most importantly, the JSS will "contribute significantly to the modern task-tailored and globally deployable combat capable forces" by meeting the replenishment and sustainment requirements of both the Canadian Naval Task Group and joint air and land based forces.[15]

Conceptually, the joint multipurpose function of the JSS is sound but, as is often the case with complex capability issues, the "devil is in the detail" when it comes to operationalizing how these concepts are going to apply and how the JSS will function in a joint operating environment. Lack of joint doctrine compounds the challenge of realizing the full extent of the JSS supporting capabilities, especially for the Army.[16] Though the Army continues to question the utility of the JSS as a result of the limited capability to lift equipment and personnel at the same time, both the Army and Air Force have committed to the conceptual utility of the JSS.[17] This conflict between conceptualization and employment is most clearly highlighted by a dichotomy between the requirement for a high readiness fleet support ship and a low readiness Army cargo ship.[18] As will be identified later in the chapter, utilizing a sea-based EAASC will impact significantly the flexibility of the JSS to be used for other tasks, such as sealift capability for forces ashore.[19] To be a truly cost-effective, multi-purpose, joint capability, the JSS must be capable of performing more than one task concurrently when deployed in all but exceptional circumstances, such as the EAASC role. Until Canadian joint doctrine is developed to explain how the JSS will be integrated into the Task Group and how the Task Group will "transport, protect and support land and air units ashore,"[20] the ability to determine the exact requirement for a JSS-based Role 3 HSS capability will prove challenging.

FUTURE BATTLESPACE

The characteristics of the post 9/11 security environment will affect the ability of the JSS to carry out a multipurpose function by placing restrictions on mobility and by increasing requirements for external force protection. The future battlespace must also be a key risk management consideration for operational planners when determining the employment of sea-based Role 3 HSS. The "inextricable relationship between events on the land and those at sea" can place the JSS in an increased threat situation, and, therefore risk the HSS capability.[21] This relationship was clearly illustrated by Commander Steve Bell when he stated that:

> Most of maritime warfare in the near term is likely to take place in coastal or littoral zones as it has for most of history. In the past, littoral zones were interpreted to be the narrow strip of water bordering a state's coast. That definition, however, has evolved to the point where littoral areas are now considered to extend from well inland out over the continental shelf and in some cases to the limits of the national economic zone… These zones create unique challenges – manoeuvre room is limited, warning times are reduced, and acoustic conditions are difficult…In this new security environment naval forces will face threats from asymmetrical weapons and forces…these are all serious threats and are extremely difficult to protect against.[22]

In these conditions, the JSS will be "a large and high value unit that is likely to be a primary target for such attacks. As a result…JS [Joint Support] vessel(s) would need adequate self-protection capability to provide warning and defence."[23] As the vast majority of the world's population lives within reach of a coastline, the ability of the JSS to operate within the littorals will place it in high demand to fulfill multiple tasks. The risk to the JSS operating in an environment characterized by unconventional strategies, as described by Bell, and the unprecedented reach and lethality of weapons, will form a key aspect of determining when sea-based Role 3 HSS can and should be utilized.

Smith summarized the threats to naval forces when he stated that "in future littoral warfare, air, sea and ground launched missiles, as well as mines and other familiar weapons, will create a tactical environment of unparalleled complexity."[24] As advances in technology are made threats, such as those from "smart mines," anti-ship missiles, torpedoes, tactical aircraft, and weapons of mass effect,[25] may result in large slow sustainment ships moving seaward to protect against an "enemy who sees sustainment as the assault forces' Achilles heel."[26] This comment is well supported by history, and can be highlighted by the experience of the Royal Navy during the Falklands conflict. Out of 23 Royal Fleet Auxiliary (RFA) vessels in theatre, six were successfully attacked by either shore-based or air-launched Exocet missiles. The mean casualty rates for both Royal Navy warships and RFA vessels averaged 8.26 sailors Killed in Action and 5.78 sailors Wounded in Action per strike.[27] Despite the brief duration of the Falklands conflict and inferior enemy capability, these rates were similar to those experienced by the US during Second World War Pacific operations. Such rates highlight both the increased risk of littoral operations and the fact that "contemporary changes to ships may not make a difference to the number of casualties sustained when an adversary is able to penetrate air defences."[28] Identifying specific threats to sea-based HSS during the operational planning process will ensure that the HSS capability will not be unduly exposed to attack and possible destruction during littoral operations.

THREATS TO SEA-BASED HSS

Protecting health services assets from attack is a fundamental aspect of HSS planning. This protection is offered under the Geneva Conventions, and, therefore International Law, for those who display the Red Cross/Crescent on HSS elements - even if it is not openly displayed.[29] For example hospital ships displaying the Red Cross/Crescent, using restricted communications, advertising the ship's location and restricting mobility indicates the non-combatant and neutral status of all personnel and assets covered. Geneva Conventions protection comes with the implicit understanding that HSS personnel and assets will not in any way aid or participate in combat.

Though HSS elements are entitled to protection, the protection will cease if the HSS elements are deemed to be committing a hostile act.[30] The JSS will *not* be a hospital ship, as defined under the Geneva Conventions and will be considered a combatant ship as a result of the multipurpose function to support combatant forces. Simply put, co-locating combat and HSS elements places the capability at increased risk of a deliberate or accidental targeting. A successful enemy strike against the JSS will not only make casualties of the ship's crew and embarked medical staff, but will potentially eliminate the only Canadian Role 3 HSS in the AO. Therefore, it is very important to explore the risks and benefits of locating a Role 3 HSS capability on this type of non-traditional, non-Geneva Conventions protected platform before deploying with this capability. While the CF has no plans to construct a hospital ship, the lessons learned from previous conflicts help to illustrate risks and benefits of sea-based Role 3 HSS in an asymmetrical threat environment.

A review of enemy action taken again Geneva Conventions-protected HSS elements on sea and land indicates that displaying the Red Cross/Crescent does not necessarily provide protection from attack, yet it may significantly restrict the movement and flexibility of HSS elements. The history of the hospital ship, which has been the backbone of traditional naval Role 3 HSS for many nations, provides an important perspective on the protective value of the Red Cross/Crescent in symmetric threat environments. Large, slow moving hospital ships, painted white and prominently marked with large Red Crosses/Crescents and afforded protected neutrality (and non-combatant status) under the Geneva Conventions have not fared well in past conflicts despite their protected status. No fewer than 28 clearly marked hospital ships were sunk during the First and Second World Wars as a result of mine and torpedo attacks.[31] Modern day examples of the protected status of the Red Cross/Crescent in asymmetric threat environments are no more favorable. During the conflict in Chechnya, insurgents deliberately targeted and destroyed soft-sided ambulances, medical posts and medical evacuation helicopters.[32] While no modern examples of deliberate targeting of clearly marked protected vessels can be found, the insurgents in Chechnya reflect one of the dangerous faces of modern asymmetrical warfare. It is reasonable to assume that hospital ships will not fare any better than their forbears in the 21st century battlespace where long-range missiles will be readily available and unconventional tactics may be used to indiscriminately inflict the greatest possible damage to Allied and coalition forces. Clearly, protected status under the Geneva Conventions is only as good as the desire of the enemy to act in accordance with international laws; in the absence of such a desire, a hospital ship could prove to be an inviting target.

Geographical separation is one of the few protective options available to Geneva Conventions-protected hospital ships in any operational scenario, and would be one of the defensive postures available to the JSS in an increased threat environment. During Operation Iraqi Freedom in 2003-4, the US Navy's hospital ship *Comfort* was located outside of the littoral AO. Evacuation of casualties to the ship proved challenging as a result of the large distances from shore-based staging facilities, dust storms and the general threat level.[33] Though Geneva Conventions-protected vessels should enjoy freedom from attack and freedom of movement, history has shown that the operational restrictions of Geneva Conventions-protected ships severely challenge the JTF Commander's ability to provide Role 3 HSS to the JTF. Lack of mobility and geographical separation, as a result of asymmetrical threats, restricted communications, and inability to return recovered troops directly to battle suggest that the concept of the hospital ship may become an anachronism of past symmetrical wars.

Understanding the risks and benefits of delivering sea-based HSS both with and without the protected status of the Geneva Conventions will allow operational planners to better manage the risk of providing JSS-based HSS for any operational planning scenario. If, as Nordick states, sea and air superiority will be secured prior to launching a land campaign, then future threats to naval forces will be significantly decreased.[34] Threats from mines, submarines and shore based missiles, however, are still difficult to eradicate. Consequently, the threat level from sea, ground and air will continue to require careful consideration prior to committing sea-based Role 3 HSS. Additional taskings, such as underway replenishment and sustainment, might necessitate that the JSS move into a position that may place the vessel within enemy weapons range in order to sustain naval combat operations. If operational commanders determine that the elevated threat level places the HSS capability at high risk despite the force protection provided to the JSS from other warships, then serious consideration must be given to moving the HSS task elsewhere. This is a costly challenge to these other JSS functions given that, generally, only one JSS will be deployed as part of a Canadian Naval Task Group at one time and "without the ability to re-supply its warships at sea, the Canadian Navy would be hard pressed to sustain a naval operation."[35]

ROLE 3 HSS OF THE FUTURE

The challenges of operating in littoral zones have caused Allied navies to rethink how to more effectively provide sea-based HSS to the sick and wounded. The realities of modern national, continental and international operations, coupled with the fiscal realities many nations are facing have resulted in innovative, risk-managed approaches to HSS delivery at all levels. Necessity has long been the catalyst in HSS evolution. In the Second World War, tank landing ships (LSTs) were converted to forward surgical ships, and later used to help control the flow of casualties to the rear. They were flexible and mobile, and proved to be relatively safe from attack despite their absence of Red Cross markings and stationing in the littoral zone.[36] One of the first Canadian examples of using a non-hospital ship to provide medical care occurred during Canadian participation in the United Nations Emergency Force during the Suez Crisis in 1956. The Canadian aircraft carrier, *HMCS Magnificent*, was equipped to "provide a small hospital to accommodate the sick and injured in the force."[37] The best example of recent HSS innovation, and a model for the current medical capabilities of the JSS, comes from the experience of the Royal Navy during the build up to Operation Desert Storm in 1990. Sea- and land-based casualty projections indicated a requirement for increased Role 3 medical capability, and the Royal Fleet Auxiliary (RFA) *Argus*, originally built as a sea training ship, was converted into a multipurpose casualty receiving ship that contained a 100 bed, Role 3 medical facility. Due to its proximity to land-based medical staging facilities, the Argus proved to be an extremely efficient in its mission. Additionally, it enjoyed protection from the naval Task Group, greatly increasing the manoeuvrability and flexibility of the platform. RFA *Argus'* successful mission was credited to the employment of a "gray hull" (non-Geneva Conventions protected) vessel.[38] The Royal

Navy's experience with the *Argus* in Iraq in 2003 proved once again that the risk of losing Geneva Conventions-protected status in favour of the manoeuvrability and relative protection of a "gray hull" was advantageous in the delivery of role 3 HSS in the context of modern conflict.[39]

The German Navy recently followed suit and completed construction of a Role 3 medical facility on the multipurpose auxiliary ship, the FGS *Berlin*.[40] It is unclear how the multipurpose functions of the *Berlin* will be impacted by the presence of a Role 3 HSS function, but it will be worth monitoring German progress as the FGS *Berlin*'s multiple sustainment, replenishment and medical capabilities most closely reflect those of the JSS. As our Allies have demonstrated, the risk of trading Geneva Conventions protection for manoeuvrability and flexibility of a combatant ship has resulted in timely access to Role 3 HSS. Employed correctly, with careful consideration given to the operational situation and appropriate risk management, Canadian sea-based joint Role 3 HSS is poised to deliver significant benefit to CF expeditionary forces.

PROVISION OF SEA-BASED HSS

The preceding discussion has focused on factors that require careful consideration prior to embedding joint Role 3 HSS within the JSS structure, and has addressed the critical force protection issues once the JSS deploys. This final part of the chapter will focus on the general concepts of HSS planning that must be considered once the commitment has been made to employ joint sea-based Role 3 HSS.[41] Adherence to these concepts will not only maximize the survivability of the sick and wounded (the key function of Force Health Protection) but will ultimately determine the degree to which the JSS will be able to carry out other roles and tasks once committed to a medical mission. Smith summarized the challenges associated with balancing competing operational requirements and effective HSS delivery as follows:

> The important question to the commander of a littoral operation is whether sea-based medical support mechanisms on hand will adequately support casualty retrieval and survival – or conversely, lead to premature death and protracted, complicated morbidity among those who survive their initial injuries.[42]

The manoeuvrability of the JSS, scalability of the medical capabilities, integral helicopter casualty evacuation capability, and the high readiness state of the JSS make adherence to HSS principles and precepts potentially easy for planners. Further, adhering to them will provide the JTF Commander with a framework to determine what other roles the JSS can perform without unduly jeopardizing Role 3 HSS.

The JSS will be a highly mobile platform designed to carry out a number of sustainment and supporting tasks to both Canadian joint and naval forces. Operationally, the JSS will provide the Joint Task Force Commander with "flexibility in decisions regarding timing and location of troop committals, and provides options in countries with non existent, poor or overburdened infrastructure."[43] The mobility of the JSS will result in the ability to deliver not only sustainment, but also early in-theatre surgical support within close proximity to the combat zone. The JSS also will possess the ability to support both sea and shore-based casualties. At present, it is unrealistic to assume that the JSS will be used as amphibious support for high intensity, high casualty land battles,[44] but as Gouge pointed out, "providing care to early casualties will be critical to mission success at the time when the medical footprint is extremely limited,"[45] and this is a task the JSS enhanced medical capability can certainly perform. However, the challenge of constructing a multipurpose ship in the absence of joint doctrine or awareness of future JSS missions may place different tasks directly in conflict with one another. While the lack of doctrine may compromise its desired capabilities once the role of the JSS is fully realized, a general lack of understanding of HSS planning factors by personnel outside of the Canadian Forces Health Services may not only impact casualty survivability and long term morbidity, but also on the ability to prioritize competing demands.[46] Therefore, joint doctrine for the JSS must be developed and agreed upon by the Army, Navy and Air Force in order to help reduce conflicting demands on the JSS capabilities once deployed.

TIMELY ACCESS TO HEALTH SERVICE SUPPORT

The concept of "humans as perishable cargo" continues to be relevant in the battlespace of the future. Many factors, such as the battle rhythm, environmental conditions, and lack of casualty evacuation assets, will significantly challenge the ability to provide timely HSS from the JSS platform. The main principle underpinning the roles of HSS delivery is that the highest role of care should be provided as close to the point of injury, commensurate with the tactical situation. The roles of HSS exist within a progressive system of casualty care that takes casualties from the point of injury to the level of care dictated by their medical status. Casualties continue to progress through the HSS system until they are ready to return to duty or be transferred out of the AO for further treatment. This stepped approach to HSS is utilized by our NATO and coalition allies, and helps to facilitate interoperability when working in a joint and combined environment. While there are variations in the terminology used to identify the roles of HSS between individual NATO and coalition allies, the capabilities remain consistent.[47] Simply put, the capabilities delivered at the different roles of Canadian HSS, in addition to the continuous and progressively more complex nature of the medical care delivered, optimize the survivability of the sick and wounded while assisting commanders to clear the battlespace by either evacuating the severely injured or returning the recovered to duty.[48] According to Smith and Llewelyn, "when a field medical system is functioning efficiently, it should be able to 'fix [treat] forward' to prevent itself from becoming a giant evacuation conduit through which experienced soldiers and marines pour out of the theatre to rear echelon health care facilities."[49] The JSS will provide a platform that can treat forward and, as it is not designated as a hospital ship, it can return the recovered directly to duty with their units. Roles of care are inextricably linked with trauma management concepts and to the timelines of evacuation from point of injury to surgical intervention, and non-medical taskings must take into account these concepts.

THE GOLDEN HOUR

The critical period of time available to deliver resuscitative HSS to battle casualties is inversely proportional to the severity of the injury. As Smith stated, "Without early medical treatment (an extremely 'time sensitive' reality) some unstable casualties will die, and the wounds of others will become seriously complicated disabilities."[50] He goes on to state that up to 20 percent of combat casualties die as a result of lack of surgical treatment for surgically correctable injuries.[51] The term "Golden Hour" has been used to define the time period when the casualty should receive initial lifesaving resuscitative trauma care. Though the term is somewhat misleading in the case of penetrating trauma, such as ballistic injuries (gunshot wounds, for example), it adequately indicates the requirement for rapid evacuation and care of the casualty.[52] The Canadian ratification draft of HSS doctrine mirrors Smith's comments in regard to the importance of urgent intervention. The doctrine has interlinked the precepts of time and evacuation, and has reinforced the concept of the "Golden Hour," going on to further indicate that the acceptable time limit to *complete* surgical intervention for non-life or limb threatening injuries is six hours.[53] The manoeuvrability of the JSS makes it an ideal platform on which to locate joint Role 3 HSS so that these treatment timelines can be met. However, JSS manoeuvrability and the requirement to multi-task the JSS has the potential to also extend the lines of casualty evacuation to a point where sea-based HSS is, in effect, no longer accessible.[54] Depending on the mission scenario, providing sea-based joint Role 3 HSS could significantly restrict the movement of the JSS and will ultimately impact either the medical task or other sustainment and replenishment functions.

EVACUATION

The most critical vulnerability of any HSS plan is the ability to evacuate casualties to and from the JSS platform.[55] From an HSS perspective, the chain of evacuation and treatment starts from the point of injury, and is directly influenced by the tactical, environmental, and geographical situation along with the extended lines of communication to be covered in a littoral environment. According to current plans, JSS-based maritime helicopters and surface boats will be made available for casualty transfer if the JSS is committed to a medical mission.[56] The availability of ships' boats, as a method of transport for casualties able to tolerate this mode of transport will greatly enhance the flexibility of the HSS plan; however, as the type of casualty most likely evacuated to the JSS will be too unstable to tolerate transport in a surface watercraft, access to tactical air medical evacuation will be essential. Additionally, if medical estimates indicate increased casualty rates, the large distances to be covered in a littoral environment require nothing less than a dedicated on-call evacuation helicopter.[57] This requirement will result in fewer helicopters being available for other taskings. The ability of the JSS to operate within the littoral zone in addition to ready, if not immediate, access to evacuation resources, will help to maintain the proximity of HSS to the point of injury. Nevertheless, if the JSS moves beyond the effective range of the maritime helicopter, access to evacuation assets will cease to be a mitigation strategy for increased distances caused by attending to other tasks, and is an issue that must be addressed prior to completing any other taskings.

The multi-layering of tasks on a limited platform may result in the inability to commit to two or more major tasks without degrading support to other. This multi-layering may prove particularly problematic for delivery of HSS if the JSS moves outside of the geographical area of land-based supported elements for a period of time deemed too long by the medical estimation process. It is likely that Canada will deploy as part of a coalition or Allied operation, but HSS planners must identify for the JTF Commander situations when multiple task commitments will result in the chain of evacuation extending beyond the six-hour surgical inter-vention window. In this case, the Task Force Surgeon must be able to designate alternate coalition Role 3 facilities to support the Task Group. This could prove to be challenging if allied or coalition partners fail to reasonably meet the Canadian standard of health care.[58] However, if no acceptable alternate sources of coalition Role 3 HSS can be found, sea-based Role 3 HSS may prove to be an operational liability and a strategic "red card" that limits the JSS's mobility and flexibility to perform other tasks.[59] Integrating the Task Force Surgeon into the JSS-based Joint Headquarters will ensure timely medical advice is given to the Joint Task Force Commander and will allow the Task Force Surgeon to exercise better operational control of all HSS assets in the JTF.[60]

Mitigating the risks to the sick and injured caused by delays in the chain of evacuation is very important in light of requirement of the JSS to provide joint, Role 3 HSS to sea- and land-based forces in some operational planning scenarios. Weger proposes a rethinking of how HSS is staged and delivered to the land forces that are equally relevant to maximize the sea-based HSS capability and to provide additional flexibility for the JSS to perform other non-medical tasks from the platform. Although a concept not yet in use in Canada, Weger advocates moving rapid surgical intervention as far forward as the tactical situation permits. In this situation, HSS would be delivered by a mobile Forward Surgical Team (FST), ideally controlled and deployed with their equipment from the JSS platform. In the current fiscally restrictive environment, it is likely that only one Canadian land- or sea-based Advanced Surgical Centre will be available within the AO at any one time.[61] Using an FST would serve, therefore, to not only make the land-based medical footprint smaller and more maneuverable, but would also ensure limited HSS resources are effectively used and services are not unnecessarily duplicated. The potential effectiveness of the FST is high-lighted by the US and UK who currently utilize FSTs. They have reduced death and disability rates of injured soldiers and sailors as a result.[62] If Canada adopts this approach, casualties will still require continued evacuation to, and treatment from, the AASC, but initial life and limb saving intervention by FSTs will have occurred earlier, thereby slightly reducing the immediate requirement for maritime helicopter evacuation capability while concurrently increasing the flexibility of the JSS for other essential tasks.

CONCLUSION

The JSS is planned to be a highly mobile platform designed to carry out a number of sustainment and supporting tasks to Canadian joint and naval forces. The JSS could prove to be the first truly joint capability available to the CF. The integrated medical capability will provide both the Navy and Joint Task Force with a level of flexibility and mobility in the provision of CF HSS that has been previously unmatched. Sea-based HSS has the potential to provide the CF with a readily deployable, scalable Role 3 HSS capability that will substantially reduce the logistical challenges presented by the relatively immobile medical footprint characterized by shore-based, Role 3 facilities. As a result of being integrated into the JSS structure, a sea-based HSS capability more easily meets the general concepts of HSS planning, particularly the requirement to meet the Canadian standard of care. As the CF's commitment to domestic, continental and international tasks increases in tempo and complexity, the availability of sea-based, joint, Role 3 HSS will be an efficient use of scarce HSS resources if HSS planners and JTF Commanders adhere to the concepts of operational HSS planning and delivery, and commit to utilizing the capability prior to construction of the first JSS.

While the JSS is, conceptually, a practical platform to deliver joint, Role 3 HSS from in the current and future littoral battlespace, protecting HSS resources from damage or destruction will be an essential consideration for Canadian JTF Commanders prior to deployment, especially as the AASC or EAASC maybe the only Canadian Role 3 facility in the AO. The asymmetric warfare tactics used by insurgents and terrorists in the post-9/11 security environment indicate that, even when carrying out a medical mission, the JSS may prove to be an inviting target to an enemy who wishes to inflict a large psychological blow to the opposing force. In such cases, force protection considerations may result in the JSS being moved seaward, which may not only impact the ability of the JSS to carry out multiple sustainment and replenishment tasks by placing restrictions on the mobility of the vessel, but the geographical separation from land-based forces will likely take the JSS beyond the six hour time limit acceptable for completing surgical interventions on the injured - a key concept of HSS.

A review of historical and current issues surrounding the delivery of sea-based joint, Role 3 HSS indicates that integrating and utilizing this capability will likely result in decreased death and disability rates of the sick and injured, as was the experience of the Royal Navy's RFA *Argus* in both Gulf Wars. The risk of placing Role 3 HSS on the JSS will need to be carefully weighed by operational planners to determine if the JSS is at an unacceptable risk of being deliberately or accidentally targeted by sea- or land-based weapons. This evaluation will need to be made prior to leaving home port as serious damage to or the sinking of the JSS has the potential to eliminate the only source of Canadian HSS in the AO.

The most critical vulnerability of any HSS plan is the ability to evacuate shore- or sea-based casualties to and from the JSS platform. The concept of timely access to care will be the key risk factor that a JTF Commander and Canadian Naval Task Group Commander will need to consider when determining what other tasks and functions the JSS will be able to complete in light of the operational scenario. As it is likely that only one JSS will be deployed at any given time, the ability to mitigate the risk of increased morbidity or mortality to the sick and injured caused by extended evacuation times, while maximizing the multipurpose function of the JSS platform, will be essential. Integrating the Task Force Surgeon into the sea-based JTFHQ to provide medical advice to the JTF Commander and Canadian Naval Task Group Commander will provide a realistic risk assessment. Introducing Forward Surgical Teams as part of the HSS package, controlled by the Task Force Surgeon and deployed from the JSS platform, will provide early life saving surgical treatment, and will provide the JSS with greater mobility and flexibility to complete other critical taskings. However, failure to address the evacuation issues surrounding shore-based casualties will render sea-based HSS capability irrelevant – or even hazardous to the casualties' survival.

Finally, the lack of comprehensive joint doctrine compounds the challenge of realizing the full extent of the JSS supporting capabilities as the multi-layering of tasks on this limited platform may result in the inability to commit to two or more major tasks without degrading support to other tasks. The challenge to effectively utilize the resource- and space-intensive medical capability will be directly impacted by the multi-purpose function of the JSS. Until comprehensive Canadian joint doctrine exists, the medical capability is at risk of being under utilized, as other JSS functions compete for primacy.

The concept of "humans as perishable cargo" continues to be relevant in the battlespace of the future. Many factors such as the battle rhythm, environmental conditions, and the access to casualty evacuation assets for transport to and from the JSS will significantly challenge the ability to provide timely HSS from the JSS platform. However, if maximally employed and carefully balanced with other JSS tasks, sea-based, joint, Role 3 HSS has the potential significantly improve the JTF Commander's ability to deliver force health protection to the Task Force while simultaneously providing sustainment and replenishment to forces on shore and at sea.

NOTES

1   A.M. Smith, "Care Delayed is Care Denied: Casualty Handling in Littoral Operations," *Naval War College Review* 52, no. 4 (Autumn 1999), 109-21.

2   Michael Gardner, Eric Dudley and David Sanschagrin, "The Joint Support Ship for the Canadian Navy – Medical Capability," presentation to the Shipboard Medical Facilities Workshop, Toulon, France, May 2004. The AOR's current medical capability can be expanded to include a limited life and limb saving surgical and post-operative care for up to four patients of varying degrees of illness and injury.

3   Canada, Department of National Defence (DND), "'Canada First' Defence Procurement - Joint Support Ship," News Release 06.030 (26 June 2006), available at http://www.forces.gc.ca/ site/newsroom/view_news_e.asp?id=1959, accessed 4 July 2006.

4   K.E. Williams, "The Canadian Navy: In the Vanguard of Canadian Foreign and Defence policy," in

Ann L. Griffiths, ed. *The Canadian Navy and the New Security Agenda: Proceedings of the Maritime Security and Defence Seminar* (Halifax, NS: Centre for Foreign Policy Studies, Dalhousie University, April 2004), 18.

5   Paul T. Mitchell, "Joint Support Ship: Transformation or White Elephant," *US Naval Institute Proceedings Proceedings of the United States Naval Institute* 130, no. 3 (March 2004), 64.

6   Role 3 is defined as the minimum capabilities of this role, including resuscitation, initial surgery, post-operative care, and short-term surgical and medical in-patient care. Diagnostic services such as x-ray and laboratory, and limited internal medicine and psychiatric services are also available. This typically includes HSS elements that are operationally responsible to a Canadian Task Force Commander (e.g., field hospital, advance surgical centers, JSS surgical centre). The Roles are described in detail in Annex C to Chapter 3 in this volume.

7   The AASC will be built into the ship and will contain one operating room and 15 beds that are able to care for both critically and seriously ill and injured patients.

8   An EAASC includes an additional operating room (OR) and 15 additional critical and intermediate care beds. These elements will be in a modularized, scalable containerized system that can be utilized on the JSS deck or taken ashore.

9   With recent changes to NATO definitions of the capabilities provided at each role, it is most likely that the enhanced JSS medical capability will be re-classed as a NATO Role 2+ facility. As the term "limited Role 3" has been used exclusively throughout the JSS project documentation, "Role 3" will be used in this paper for consistency.

10   Captain (N) Jung, former Chief of Maritime Staff Medical Advisor and architect of the JSS medical capability, in a conversation with the author 5 October 2004. He stated that the AASC will be an HSS asset utilized for all sea-, land- and air-based CF troops in the AO, reflecting the joint nature of sea-based HSS.

11   Mitchell, "Joint Support Ship," 64.

12   DND, *Health Services Support to Canadian Forces Operations (Ratification Draft)*, B-GJ-005-410/FP-000 (Ottawa: DND, 2004), p. 1-5.

13   David Salisbury and Allan English, "Prognosis 2020: A Military Medical Strategy for the Canadian Forces," *Canadian Military Journal* 4, no.2 (Summer 2003), 47.

14   Mitchell, "Joint Support Ship," 65.

15   DND, *Statement of Operational Requirements* (Ottawa: Project Management Office Joint Support Ship DSP 2673, May 2004), 2.

16   Ann L. Griffiths, "Summary of Plenary Discussion: The Navy and Canada's New Security Agenda," in Griffiths, ed. *The Canadian Navy and the New Security Agenda*,106.

17   Steve Bell, "The Naval Strategic Plan," in Griffiths, ed. *The Canadian Navy and the New Security Agenda*, 66.

18   Robert H. Edwards, "The Future of Canada's Maritime Capabilities: The Issues, Challenges and Solutions in a New Security Environment 18-20 June 2004: Conference Report," rough draft provided by the Centre for Foreign Policy Studies, Dalhousie University, Halifax, 34.

19   DND, *Statement of Operational Requirements*, Annex A, p.18.

20   Edwards, "The Future of Canada's Maritime Capabilities," 36.

21   Arthur M. Smith, "The Influence of Medicine on Strategy," *Naval War College Review* 41, no. 2 (Spring 1988), 26.

22   Bell, "The Naval Strategic Plan," in Griffiths, ed. *The Canadian Navy and the New Security Agenda*, 72-3.

23   DND, *Statement of Operational Requirements*, 12

24   Smith. "Care Delayed is Care Denied," 2.

25   Bell, "The Naval Strategic Plan," in Griffiths, ed. *The Canadian Navy and the New Security Agenda*, 73.

26   Smith, "Care Delayed is Care Denied," 2.

27   Christopher G. Blood, et al., "Casualty Incidence during Naval Combat Operations: A Matter of Medical Readiness," *Naval War College Review* 49, no. 4 (Autumn 1996), 4.

28   Ibid., 3.

29   In the case of an enemy boarding on a warship, the HSS facility should not be attacked or destroyed despite its location on the warship. In this instance, the Red Cross symbol would not displayed external to the ship, but would be easily identified once on board.

30   DND, *The Law of Armed Conflict at the Operational and Tactical Level – Annotated*, B-GG-005-027/AF-021 (Ottawa: Office of the Judge Advocate General, 2001), 17-5. An HSS facility is deemed to be committing a hostile act if it is, or appears to be, aiding the war effort of one side.

31   Smith, "Care Delayed is Care Denied," 5.

32   L.W. Grau and T.L.Thomas, "'Soft Log' and Concrete Canyons: Russian Urban Combat Logistics in Grozny," *Marine Corps Gazette* 83, no. 10 (October1999), 67-75.

33   Captain Allington, US Navy, CO USNS COMFORT, personal communication with the author, 18 August 2004; and Grau and Thomas, "'Soft Log' and Concrete Canyons," 67- 76.

34   G. Nordick, "Can the CF Develop Viable National Joint Capabilities?" *Canadian Military Journal* 5, no. 2 (Summer 2004), 62-7.

35   DND, "Canada's Navy: News and Information—Issues and Challenges. The Value of Canada's Replenishment Ships," http://www.navy.forces.gc/mpsa_news_issues_e.asp?category=2&title=16, accessed 19 Oct 2004.

36   Smith, "Care Delayed is Care Denied," 6.

37   DND, *Canadian Participation in the United Nations Emergency Force*, Report No. 94 Historical Section Army Headquarters (Ottawa: DND, 1961), 24.

38   Smith, "Care Delayed is Care Denied," 7.

39   Robert Fox, *Iraq Campaign 2003 Royal Navy and Royal Marines* (London: Agenda Publishing, 2003), 131.

40   Observations during a visit to the FGS *Berlin* by the author in May 2004.

41   DND, *Health Services Support to Canadian Forces Operations (Ratification Draft)*, pp. 1-5, 1-6. The principles that guide HSS planning are conformity, proximity flexibility, mobility, continuity and control. The precepts of HSS planning outline the 12 legal, policy and/or operational imperatives that must be considered.

42   Smith, "Care Delayed is Care Denied," 1.

43   Greg Aikens, "Beyond ALSC: We Need to get Amphibious and Joint to Stay Relevant," *Maritime Affairs Newsletter* (Winter 2001), 12-13, available at http://atoz.ebsco.com, accessed 24 September 2004.

44   Mitchell, "Joint Support Ship," 66; and Edwards, "The Future of Canada's Maritime Capabilities," 34.

45   S.F. Gouge, *Combat Health Support of the Transformation Force in 2015*, (Carlisle Barracks, PA: US Army War College, 2001), 21.

46   Edwards, "The Future of Canada's Maritime Capabilities," 35.

47   US Department of Defense (DoD), *Doctrine for Health Service Support in Joint Operations*, Joint Publication 4-02 (Washington: DoD, 2001); United Kingdom, Department of Defence, *United Kingdom Doctrine for Joint and Multinational Operations (Interim Edition)*, Joint Warfare Publication 0-10 (London: Ministry of Defence, n.d), 8-11; and DND, *Health Services Support to Canadian Forces Operations (Ratification Draft)*, pp. 1-7, 1-8.

48   To find a detailed description of the capabilities found at the 4 roles of HSS, see DND, *Health Services Support to Canadian Forces Operations (Ratification Draft)*, pp. 1-7, 1-8.

49   A.M. Smith and C.H. Llewellyn, "Caring for our Casualties," *US Naval Institute Proceedings* 117, no. 12 (December 1991), 72-8.

50   Smith, "Care Delayed is Care Denied," 1.

51   A.M. Smith, "All Bleeding Stops Eventually," *US Naval Institute Proceedings* 127, no. 11 (November 2001), 68.

52   G. Cecchine, et al., *Army Medical Support to the Army After Next : Issues and Insights from the Medical Technology Workshop*, 1999 (Santa Monica: RAND, 2000), 18.

53   DND, *Health Services Support to Canadian Forces Operations (Ratification Draft)*, p. 2-6.

54   The JSS Statement of Requirement document has acknowledged that TG support may not be compatible with other taskings if it does not possess the necessary freedom of movement.

55   Smith, "Care Delayed is Care Denied," 3.

56   It is planned to have four Maritime Helicopters attached to each JSS. HSS planning indicates rearward to forward movement of medical evacuation assets meaning that receiving facilities normally move forward to pick up casualties. DND, *Statement of Operational Requirements*, Annex A.

57   Smith, "Care Delayed is Care Denied," 3.

58   DND, *Health Services Support to Canadian Forces Operations (Ratification Draft)*, p. 2-6. Regardless of the geographical location, "the levels of health care shall be provided at levels of accessibility and quality comparable to those being afforded to Canadians, in general." NATO Allied Joint Medical Support Doctrine, US Joint Doctrine, and UK Joint Doctrine contain similar statements, reflecting similar emphasis being placed on robust HSS for expeditionary forces.

59   The provision of HSS to CF expeditionary operations is inextricably linked to strategic and political priorities and realities. Health care is the number one priority for Canadians and boards of inquiry, such as the Croatia Board of Inquiry, have articulated why robust HSS is critical to success of the mission at all levels - at the tactical/operational interface to conserve fighting strength and at the strategic/political interface to ensure that the CF maintains the support and commitment of the Canadian public. See DND, *Final Report: Board of Inquiry - Croatia* (Ottawa: DND, 2000).

60   Capt (N) Jung, telephone conversation with the author 5 October 2003.

61   Ibid.

62   David Weger, "Blurring of the Lines: The Call for an Integrated Surgical Capability in Canadian Field Ambulances," paper written for the Advanced Military Studies Course, Canadian Forces College (2003), 24. Weger's paper is Chapter 4 in this volume.

CHAPTER 8

CFHS HEAL THYSELF: DEVELOPING STRATEGIC HEALTH SERVICES LEADERS FOR THE MODERN MILIEU

Colonel James C. Taylor

[Strategic leaders] must understand the operational imperative of their mission, but they must also understand the other key aspects of it, even if these may be less dramatic or less appealing …credibility, visibility, accountability, responding to the effect of changes in society, and interfacing with politicians, civilians and the media. [1]

General (retired) John de Chastelain,
former Chief of the Defence Staff

INTRODUCTION

Current Canadian Forces Health Services (CFHS) leaders must function in a situational milieu that is significantly more complex than that of our forebears because the knowledge and skill sets that made for highly successful leaders during the Cold War are no longer sufficient in today's leadership environment. The author's generational cohort of CFHS leaders has been perhaps the most significantly impacted by the sea change in leadership that overtook the Canadian Forces (CF) in the 1990s, having spent their developmental years as junior leaders in one leadership climate, and their senior leadership years in another. The author's direct involvement in these events as they unfolded spawned his interest in leadership and leader development in the CFHS organization.

One result of this interest was a research project, described here, that sought to answer the question: How can the CFHS build a sustainable strategic leadership capacity that can operate successfully in the fluidity of our modern environment? Its associated sub-questions were:

1. What are the leader competencies required in the 21st century battlespace?
2. What are the current best practices in developing those competencies?
3. What objective processes can the CFHS use to develop those competencies in its own leaders?

This research project involved considering one of the key requirements, namely strategic leader development, for the sustainability of an organization that has undergone significant internal transformational change in recent years. This change has involved not only the structure, but also the culture of the organization, and numerous departures from the traditional roles of the subcultural groups that comprise it. One must then add to these developments the foil of change that has taken place in both the CF at large, as well as in the global military and civilian communities. These factors considered, the challenges of providing relevant and sustainable strategic leadership in the CFHS are many and varied. It is critical that the CFHS embrace new and effective leader development practices or it risks a partial or full reversal of the transformational change that has driven the CFHS in meeting its mission of promoting health protection and delivering quality care to the CF, anytime, anywhere.

Firstly, as the CFHS competes to be an employer of choice within a shrinking target recruiting demographic, along with the changes in the education, expectations and perspectives of Canadian society in specific and global society in general, leadership approaches have evolved from an authoritarian and transactional model to a participative and transformational model. Further, with the change in role from preparing to be a front line participant in a continental "force on force" mission model in northern Europe, to the current "asymmetric force" mission model for peacemaking and peacekeeping around the world, the required intellectual and social skill set model that defines the required capacities of an effective leader has changed. Superimpose on this complex milieu the technologically-, legally- and politically-charged environment that has blurred the lines between the strategic and tactical levels of operations, and it becomes readily apparent that a new paradigm of identifying, developing and empowering the strategic leadership of the CFHS must be created.

The work described in this chapter applied qualitative research methods to explore a variety of complementary sources, venues and schools of thought, and sought to synthesize a preliminary road map to the future that would assist in the assessment, development and learning of others as they prepare themselves, and are prepared by the organization, to meet the challenges of providing a sustainable CFHS strategic leadership capacity. Following an overview of the related literature on competencies and best practises, qualitative data was gathered on these two areas using a structured interview tool. The interview participant cohort comprised senior CF officers and DND academics with expertise in the area of leadership. Individual responses were combined and themed to produce the first-order data, which was then compared to the literature; a draft CFHS strategic leader development framework was then synthesized from these data. A focus group tool was then employed, involving an external facilitator and an internal CFHS participant cohort, to review the draft framework. Group responses were themed to produce the second-order data, which was then related back to the literature to produce the final framework. For reasons of brevity, the full literature review and the detailed research methodology are not presented here.[2]

The aim of this project was to continue the organizational discussion on a longstanding issue from a fresh and informed perspective, producing an innovative way ahead to be considered for implementation by the CF Health Services Group Commander. This project has produced a conceptual leader development model for the future that is designed to meet the needs of CFHS and that is a more systematic and evidence-based approach than has been used in the past. The model can contribute to the development of organizational expertise, in the areas identified, of potential strategic leaders and their subsequent and appropriate development through the processes of succession planning, training, education and mentoring. The model can also be used to replace historical CFHS leader development practices that have been recognized officially as no longer appropriate to contemporary challenges. Naturally, in a research activity of limited scope and duration such as this one, it was not the author's goal to attempt to produce a comprehensive treatise on leadership competencies and/or development practices; these exist elsewhere. The focus of this work was to establish a sufficient knowledge base, through a selective overview of the associated literature, to ask a credible question of reasonable scope on behalf of the CFHS organization, and then to apply a reasonably rigorous qualitative research process involving both internal and external stakeholders in order to produce an organizationally-derived outcome of reasonable validity. Hence, while the core of this work was the organizationally-focused and people-oriented opinion data provided and evaluated by participants with the appropriate expertise and a genuine interest in its outcome, the production of this data was guided by, accented, and considered in the context of the selected references in the literature. The outcome, in the form of a series of general recommendations, should thus be relevant to CFHS in its efforts to improve its leader development practices. The results and conclusions of the study are summarized briefly next to provide the reader with context for the discussion that follows.

STUDY RESULTS AND CONCLUSIONS

> It became clear to me that at the age of 58, I would have to learn new tricks that were not taught in the military manuals or on the battlefield. In this position I am a political soldier and will have to put my training in rapping out orders and making snap decisions on the back burner, and have to learn the arts of persuasion and guile. I must become an expert in a whole new set of skills.[3]

> General George Marshall, former Chief of Staff of the US Army

Study Findings

For reasons of brevity, the entire body of analyzed first-order data, namely the themed data from the external interviews, is not presented here; nor is the analyzed second-order data, contained in the Focus Group Report. They are available upon request. There, however, three overarching themes from the first-order interview data that must be briefly discussed here as they set the tone for the development of the conclusions.

CF Officers First. The idea that CFHS colonels should have strategic-level competencies in common with other CF colonels was a common theme among interview participants: "CFHS colonel competencies at the strategic level should be similar to those of colonels in other branches of the CF ... [and they] should receive the same training and education as line officers, plus professional training beyond that."[4] This quote speaks to the expectation that, while CFHS officers' tactical-level technical competencies (operational health care) will likely differ from those of direct combatant ("line") officers in a number of areas, they must still be CF officers before being technical specialists. This situation is not unprecedented in the CF, as there are significant differences in technical/tactical competencies even amongst line officers across the three environments.

It was suggested by another interview participant that this similarity in strategic competencies be in both "quality and depth." Further, given the CFHS rank structure and frequent global reach of activities, it was suggested that CFHS officers may need to develop and employ these competencies "at one rank lower" than other CF officers.[5] Therefore, this research is focused on the command stream, and on those CFHS officers capable of developing and successfully employing both clinical (and clinical administrative) *and* command competencies.

Operations has Primacy. A nearly universal theme amongst interview participants was that CFHS leaders "must understand what the warfighting effort is all about."[6] The issue raised here is, given that operations is the "main line of our CF business,"[7] one must understand them in depth to have "credibility" as a CF colonel.[8] The CF cultural overlay to these sentiments that has taken place during the last 10-15 years involves the refocusing of the organization away from military bureaucracy as an end unto itself, and toward the *raison d'être* for the CF - to conduct operations. The impact on the CFHS of this transformation has been a sharpened focus on health care support to CF operations.

Military Ethos. "Our bottom line is written in blood – theirs isn't."[9] This opinion represents the shared position of interview participants that, while civilian corporate practices should be studied and understood, and selected practices perhaps modified and incorporated into CF strategic leader development, it is inappropriate to adopt them wholesale, given the vastly differing missions of the two organizational communities. Indeed, it was felt that the environment in which a CF strategic-level leader must function is more complex than that of a civilian corporate CEO.[10] Sharpe and English have discussed this issue in detail,[11] and these sentiments were unequivocally shared by interview participants, who contrasted the corporate versus military models: "they seek efficiency for profits, the CF seeks effectiveness in mission outcomes." [12]

Study Conclusions. The conclusion of this study is presented graphically at Figure 8-1, and the substantiating discussion will be organized around the structure of that graphical representation.

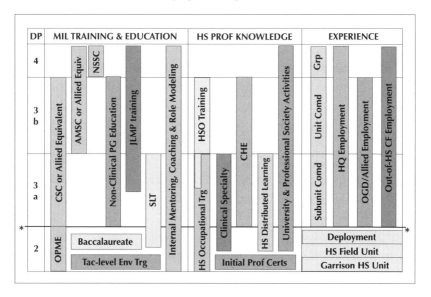

FIGURE 8-1. CFHS LEADER DEVELOPMENT FRAMEWORK

The initial idea for developing this data in three domains (i.e., military training and education, health service professional knowledge, and experience) came from a discussion in the interviews on the development procedural model of the "education, experience and training triad,"[13] where "each is necessary but not sufficient."[14] The model also serves to "map out training, professional development …, and experience" in order to develop the required competencies, employing an adult education model comprising "both experiential and formal learning" in the development of military strategic leaders.[15] Furthermore, the model is also in keeping with the US military practice of requiring a "prescribed set of experiences" for many of its senior positions.[16] Interview data suggests, with regard to elements of the triad, that education provides "critical thinking and the ability to reason" and "the ability to extrapolate from many sources to find solutions for which one was not necessarily specifically trained,"[17] and that training provides immediate "vicarious experience early and gives junior personnel the tools with which to develop their experiences." [18]

Therefore, given the "dual competencies,"[19] comprising both general CF knowledge and Health Services (HS) professional knowledge required of CFHS officers, the domains of Military Training and Education, HS Professional Knowledge, and Experience were created, comprising the overarching groups of the columnar vertical elements of the graphic matrix. The elements in the rows represent activities in three of the four CF officer Developmental Periods (DPs) designed to prepare leaders for progressively more challenging roles.[20] While it may seem odd to discuss DP 2 in a study focused on developing DP 4 officers, DP 2 is where the foundation is laid in this iterative development process as strategic leader aspirants learn the fundamentals of the "core business knowledge"[21] of the CFHS and the "tactical, technical and technological proficiency"[22] they will need to be able to "interact and engage effectively at all of the tactical, operational and strategic levels"[23] as a strategic leader, while retaining the technical competencies in order to "meet the mission on the ground."[24] Indeed, in the modern milieu, junior officers now need to grasp the potential strategic impact of their actions at the tactical level.[25] This development process is "sequential and progressive,"[26] and Guillot has reminded us that "shortcuts do not exist, and one can't start at the top."[27] This process is also in keeping with the American Productivity and Quality Center (APQC) recommendations, whereby this level of training is normally conducted and/or coordinated at the local/unit level in order to build job-related technical competencies which serve not only to support the unit tactical-level missions, but also as a foundation for future higher-level learning for the individual.[28] It is this foundation training, education and experience that readies a member for consideration within the succession-planning process at the national headquarters level.

The line between DP 2 and DP 3 represents the beginning of the CFHS succession planning process, whereby on entering DP 3 CFHS personnel are assessed against published competencies to identify the cadre of individuals with the capacity and motivation for senior leadership positions as part of the CFHS process to "grow leaders" from within.[29] This process is directly in keeping with three more of the APQC recommendations.[30] While the CFHS practices "broadly-based leader development," as called for in *Leadership in the Canadian Forces*,[31] for all

CFHS personnel by challenging all leaders with increasing responsibility and complexity of tasks throughout their careers in accordance with demonstrated competencies, its process to develop senior leaders is in line with the remainder of the CF and corporate best practices,[32] whereby succession planning processes are used to select high-potential leaders for entry into the strategic leader development process since "not all can be put through formal training."[33] The military training and education developmental activities that contribute to the strategic leader development process will be discussed next by selected domains and elements.

Military Training and Education

Baccalaureate. The requirement for CF officers to hold a baccalaureate degree is specifically endorsed by policy,[34] and would serve as an entry-level element in the development of the "mental agility" metacompetency of Wong et al.[35] References to this level of education and, by extension, to that of prior secondary matriculation, were limited in the civilian corporate literature, namely Fulkerson's requisite educational element for global executives of a "humanities or engineering degree" and a graduate degree.[36] This lack of references is attributed to the current presumption by corporations, particularly in North America, that candidates for executive-level positions will automatically arrive with at least an undergraduate degree, and most likely a subsequent graduate degree. This element was left out of the draft framework considered by the Focus Group, as it was assumed that it would be considered as a baseline activity by this group. However, given its specific inclusion in CF policy, it was included in the final framework.

Tactical-level Environmental Training. Interview participants expressed a the view that strategic leaders needed to have "tactical- and operational-level expertise"[37] as the tactical/technical foundation for their strategic leadership competencies, and that such leaders must be able to readily and rapidly shift their perspectives to "interact and engage effectively at all of the tactical, operational and strategic levels."[38] This tactical- and operational-level expertise also comprises one of the systemic domains for which organizational-level leaders are responsible within their requisite "system of systems" perspective, and it enhances their indirect leadership credibility (and therefore effectiveness) within the tactical-level elements of their organization.[39] In the CF, such knowledge is most effective when it is undertaken in each of the three CF environments, thus eventually leading to a truly "joint" perspective at the strategic level of leadership. It is also to be noted that this element is not specifically prescriptive, as there are a number of training opportunities at this level in each of the three environments that would satisfy this element of the framework. This element generated significant discussion amongst Focus Group participants, and while supportive, participants expressed concerns with regard to the perceived historic lack of universal accessibility of such training to all CFHS officer professional communities. However, as the validity of this element did not appear to be in question, it was not amended.

Second Language Training. This element requires little discussion, as CF officers are required to hold a certain profile of competency in their second official language. At the strategic level, however, this element is also supported conceptually both by the observation of Paquet et al that it enables the CF strategic leader to better reflect Canada's culture and values both domestically and internationally, and by Fulkerson's work which suggested a requirement for civilian global executives to "speak more than one language" as an intellectual competency element.[40] Second language training (SLT) is listed as a requirement in both DP 2 and DP 3A as it is accessible to CF personnel locally on their own initiative, and will improve their scores when they are assessed during the succession planning process. Limited opportunities for full-time off-site training are also available, but this costly training should logically be limited to those officers, identified through the succession planning process, who require further development in this area. It is also to be noted that, if the CFHS is to embody the spirit of the 1988 Official Languages Act and meet the requirements of current DND policy, this competency should be achieved prior to DP 3B, such that it has become integral to potential strategic leaders' competencies well before their accession to those roles, and not treated as a superficially/temporarily-grasped last-minute tick-in-the-box for which an individual takes no personal responsibility. Focus Group participants, while directly supportive of this element, expressed concern regarding the availability of access of language training to all CFHS officers, and the logistics of providing this training to the DP 2 demographic was also questioned. However, since, as described above, part-time or short-term SLT opportunities are available to all CFHS officers at the local level on their own initiative and that the limited number of full-time SLT positions would likely be specifically identified for high-potential DP 3A officers via the succession planning process, this element was not amended. It is also to be noted that all CF officers now receive an introductory period of full-time SLT in DP 1.

CF Professional Military Education. Interview participants' strong sense that CFHS colonels require, beyond their health care leadership competencies, the same common DP-related competencies as CF line officers was discussed previously. These common competencies would ensure that CFHS leaders fully comprehended the fit of the CFHS within the CF as an organization, and understood "the CF planning and decision-making processes."[41] They would also serve to enable senior CFHS leaders in their role of establishing and maintaining engagement with the political level of the national security community.[42] Such military institutional education was identified as a key element in a survey of US General Officers regarding their most important developmental experiences.[43] The published approach of the CF to the military education (i.e., Officer Professional Military Education (OPME), the Command and Staff Course (CSC), the Advanced Military Studies Course (AMSC), and the National Security Studies Course (NSSC) associated with the stepwise development of CF officers at the various DP levels, which is parallel to that practiced in the US military services, was also discussed previously. It is to be noted that OPME (normally DP 2) is available to all CF officers locally on their own initiative, and will serve to improve their scores when they are assessed during the succession planning process. Opportunities for CFHS positions on the CSC, AMSC and NSSC are limited, and should thus logically be assigned to high-potential officers identified through the succession planning process. Furthermore, positions on equivalent courses in Allied nations are available to the CF, and should be sought by the CFHS to broaden the perspectives of its future strategic leaders by developing their cross-cultural savvy metacompetency as identified by Wong et al.[44]

Non-Clinical Postgraduate Education. The non-clinical postgraduate education element is intended to develop the boundary-transcending advanced and flexible "cognitive capacities," as outlined in the discussion of education versus training above and called for by interview participants, as well as others.[45] This element supports the required competencies of creativity and innovation, and allows individuals to "expand [their] intellectual horizons"[46] to develop the breadth of perspective necessary for senior leaders to "navigate outside one's culture."[47] While interview participants all supported non-clinical postgraduate education in general and its contribution to critical thinking skills, as practiced by the American and British militaries, opinion was mixed as to whether this education should be achieved through MA, MBA or MPA programs. The only specific opinions expressed in this regard were that CFHS officers would best achieve interpersonal skills development "through exposure to the social sciences," as well as graduate education in "public sector management"[48] in preparation for strategic-level positions. A caveat was also expressed, however, that the CFHS should avoid "diploma mills"[49] and actively seek programs that will support the CFHS's environment of critical thinking and broad inquiry as a learning organization.[50] Given the time and resource investment required by such opportunities, those interviewed felt they should be assigned to high-potential officers identified by the succession-planning process, and are thus logically undertaken during the DP 3A or DP 3B stages. Given that such individuals are also normally assigned to demanding primary positions during DP 3, it is recommended that such programs, unless specifically targeted as workplace-integrated programs, be undertaken on a full-time basis so as not to degrade the richness of the residential educational experience as described by Smith.[51] It is to be noted, however, that MA programs are also available to qualified officers, on their own initiative, on a part-time distance-learning basis through RMC as previously described.

Joint, Interagency, Multinational and Public Sector (JIMP) Training. In a Canadian context, the term Joint, Interagency, Multinational and Public Sector (JIMP), "joint" means effective functional integration among the land, sea and air elements of an armed force; "interagency" means the effective interaction of an armed force with non-military bodies existing within its operating environment; "multinational" means the effective functional interaction of a national military force with the military forces of one or more friendly nations; and "public sector" means the functional coordination of DND with other Canadian government departments (OGDs) and bodies. Interview participants all supported a requirement for the development of competencies in these areas, emphasizing the necessity for a "globally aware" strategic leader to function across boundaries in the national and international political environment, successfully "interfac[ing] with government" and grasping both its published and unpublished policies and processes and how the CF "fits into the broad-er world" from a systems perspective.[52] This is in keeping with Chilcoat's recommended practice for strategic leaders of "continuous but critical 'looking outward'"[53] and Magee's strategic leader task to manage "joint, combined [which means multinational], and interagency relationships"[54] by effectively "secur[ing] the cooperation of organizations and personalities beyond one's direct influence and control."[55]   The JIMP perspective is also championed by Wong et al and Flowers as an effective contextual lens for the strategic leader and a means to extend influence, and comprises one of Smith's five key dimensions of strategic leadership.[56] Although education is normally favoured over training at the strategic level, interview participants indicated that specific training for the assimilation of new JIMP skills was effective in some areas, such as media techniques and public policy. There are a great number of national and international training opportunities at this level in each of the four areas that would contribute to competencies in this element of the framework. Hence, this is one of the elements of the Framework that will perpetually evolve and the CFHS must constantly monitor the environment to add new, relevant opportunities and to discontinue those historically-accessed opportunities which may have been rendered less relevant by the constant progression of JIMP dynamics. It is also to be noted that this element of the Framework must commence prior to DP 3B, to ensure a JIMP-focused conceptual foundation for future senior leaders, and must continue for the remainder of their careers. Focus Group participants expressed support for this element, and echoed the recommendation not to initiate it only at the DP 3B level, because it should be started earlier in the developmental periods, i.e., the senior DP 3A point.

Internal Mentoring, Coaching & Role Modeling. The importance of eth-ical and moral standards of conduct was a key theme expressed by inter-view participants, and it was emphasized that these qualities must be internalized during one's development as an officer, and not simply "'memorized' when one reaches a senior rank."[57] Wong et al recommend that these professional qualities of an officer, as well as the officer's inter-personal maturity, are best developed through role modeling and mentor-ship by the most senior personnel in the organization.[58] This approach is further supported by the survey of US General Officers, which reported that mentorship was the second most important developmental experi-ence in the success of their careers.[59] While one interview participant recommended the executive coaching models used by corporate executives, the preponderance of opinion held that formal or organizationally-assigned mentoring programs should be avoided, and that mentoring is a chain of command activity wherein "it is incumbent upon the individual to seek out appropriate mentors."[60] It was also recommended that, for CFHS officers in clinical occupations, they seek one mentor for their command development and one for their clinical development. Hence, in the CFHS Medical community, personnel might seek a clinical mentor through the professional/technical chain and command mentorship through the chain of command; in the CFHS Dental community, of course, these chains are one and the same, and all mentoring in both areas can thus be sought through the individual's chain of command. In any case, it is a chain of command responsibility to ensure that an organizational climate is fostered that supports mentorship and coaching, and it is incumbent upon CFHS senior leaders to ensure that they are effective role models and that they are living the ethos for developing officers,[61] thereby demonstrating their own competency of "reinforcing growth in others."[62] This competency would naturally include the leader's responsibility to both empower and challenge developing leaders through the appropriate delegation of authority.[63]

Besides military training and education developmental activities, for HSS senior officers, health services knowledge is a critical aspect of the strategic leader development process, and it will be discussed by element next.

Health Services Knowledge

Initial Professional Certifications. In any CF officer occupation, but particularly within the highly specialized area of health care, one's professional credentials (beyond one's generic qualifications as a CF officer), be they clinical licensure or administrative certifications, are a key foundational element of one's qualifications; further, they are part of the CFHS's benchmarking strategy to the Canadian civilian standard of health care. While these credentials are often achieved in DP 1, they are shown in the DP 2 portion of the framework to remind the senior leadership of the fundamental nature of this aspect of CFHS senior leader development. Interview participants felt that the first element of military expertise is "credibility within one's own field," in this case health care. They also emphasized the importance of professional ideology within one's own occupation as a CF officer, and how an officer's actions "must be rooted in a professional ethos."[64] This is supported by CFLI's identification of professional cohesion as an important supporting condition for strategic leader development, and represents an enabling activity for the exercise of stewardship over the profession of military health care.[65]

Health Services Occupation Training and Health Services Operations Training. Each of the occupations within the CFHS, be it clinical or administrative, has its own training elements, which are at times undertaken as common elements with other CFHS occupations. This training is principally provided at the CF Health Services Training Centre (CFHSTC), which has conformed for the last few decades to the recommendations of both APQC and Day and Halpin for a dedicated off-site leader development environment where the organization can closely control the content and delivery of learning.[66] While all CFHS occupations undergo basic tactical-level training in CFHS operations, only one occupation, Health Services Operations Officer, goes on to undertake operational-level health services operations (HSO) training, usually in DP 3A. It is important to emphasize that all CFHS occupations should undertake this HSO training, be it in DP 3A or DP 3B. This is well supported by the previous discussion on the primacy of operations in the CF, and the need to incorporate this operational focus as a requisite competency for CFHS strategic leaders to establish "credibility" with their line officer colleagues and to ensure a "broad [and shared] understanding among the [CFHS] senior cadre team" in this fundamental CF capability.[67] This premise is further supported by the Conference Board's defined essential capability for the strategic leader to grasp the "core business knowledge" of the organization, and operational health care is indeed the core business of the CFHS.[68]

Clinical Specialty Training. The inclusion of clinical specialty training here is intended to remind the CFHS senior leadership that clinical specialists as a group must not to be limited to "clinical track" roles purely by dint of their clinical credentials. The practices of our Allies and the civilian medical and dental clinical communities in Canada show that clinical specialists with the appropriate qualifications and credibility are often in top strategic leadership positions. For example, in the US Army, at least the last five Surgeons-General/Commanders of Medical Command (the strategic leader of the medical community), and at least the last five Chiefs of the Dental Corps (the strategic leader of the dental community), have been certified specialists in a discipline of medicine and dentistry respectively.[69] Further, one must take into account the strategic-level leadership practices in the civilian medical and dental clinical communities in Canada. While strategic leadership positions in both organizations and academe in Canada and the US are filled by both generalists and specialists, based on a generic skill set, national leadership in the component disciplines comprising these professions is invariably provided by certified specialists within that discipline. As the CFHS expects its strategic leaders to have influence with national decision-making bodies, and to show stewardship of the profession in the national arena by extending influence beyond chains of command, this is a component competency that cannot be ignored in building an effective CFHS senior leader team.[70]

Certified Health Executive Program. The Certified Health Executive (CHE) program certifies that an individual has achieved the core competencies for executive-level leaders in Canada's health care system. It is indeed a strategic-level leader qualification, as it transcends the individual health care professions and the military and civilian communities and focuses on the overarching system of systems in Canadian health care; as such it represents Wong's professional astuteness writ large.[71] Further, it represents Chilcoat's strategic role of "looking outwards to constantly seek wisdom from other relevant systems.[72] Although they did not identify such a program by name, interview participants supported the concept of a requisite awareness, for strategic CFHS leaders, of all of the elements of the system of systems that is Canadian health care. Ensuring that the CFHS senior leader cadre holds this qualification would give the CF further standing in the national medical community from which to foster national-level relationships which would give the CF influence with the national decision-making bodies that set the course for national medical care in Canada.[73] Unfortunately, a similar qualification for the executive management of dental organizations does not exist per se, as Canadian dentistry is largely non-institutional, being principally private-practice based.

The inclusion of this element was supported by Focus Group participants, with the caveat that participatory vigilance would have to be exercised in collaboration with the Canadian College of Health Service Executives (CCHSE) to ensure that their evaluation processes truly represented their published competency foundation.

Health Services Distributed Learning. The health services distributed learning element is intended to provide ready access to the knowledge that, while required, is not available through any of the other elements; it is thus the catch-all for didactic training gaps in the framework. It would be undertaken much as the distributed-learning mechanism of the Joint Medical Executive Skills Program (JMESP), but limited to areas of knowledge identified by the CFHS senior leadership.[74] This is in keeping with the APQC best practices of "knowledge dissemination" and "personal access to the company's knowledge capital" through technology.[75] While the value of residential full-time training and education is recognized, particularly at higher levels, distance-learning strategies for CFHS foundational leadership and management knowledge could provide organizational training "leverage."[76] Such a program could either be developed by the CFHSTC or, if the technology requirement exceeded its capability, the CFHS could seek partnership with the Canadian Defence Academy (CDA) for this initiative.

This program could be available to all CFHS officers locally (on-line) to take on their own initiative, as a recorded self-development activity, and it would improve their scores when they are assessed during the succession planning process. To ensure that this program was not seen as a typical more-with-less initiative that often engenders resentment, officers could register for the program with a learning contract that included an approved timeline. Participants would then be accorded one-half day per week for the duration of the learning contract to undertake this activity within their normal workplace during normal duty hours. Health services distributed learning received support from Focus Group participants, with the proviso that it would need significant developmental work to capture the current learning needs of CFHS officers.

University and Professional Society Activities. There was significant support for an element based on university and professional society activities amongst interview participants as it was felt that CFHS officers must know their professions through participation in clinical practice (or clinic administration for non-clinicians), through university teaching and through participation in professional associations.[77] These activities would satisfy the "need to be exposed to other worlds/communities to expand thinking"[78] and enable strategic CFHS leaders in their requisite ability to "see the next major conceptual horizon" in health care as it applies to the CF.[79] Such activities also give participating individuals the knowledge and perspective to constantly validate CFHS policies and practices, and they give the CFHS the sort of visibility and credibility to maintain the confidence that the Canadian public has in it as a world-class military health service. Further, they will give the CFHS further avenues of influence with national decision-making bodies in health care, and expand the CFHS's conceptual horizons as a learning organization in military health care.[80] Beyond the organizational benefits of these practices, the personal development aspect of this element for strategic leaders must not be underestimated.[81]

Experience. In the strategic leader development process, experience cannot be considered in isolation. It must be well coordinated with associated training and education activities, as described in the previous two domains, if the desired learning outcome is to be achieved. While not all elements will necessarily give a profound depth of expertise in any given area, all will contribute significantly to the "breadth of expertise" required of strategic leaders,[82] and contribute to meeting the requirement for CFHS colonels "to have a sense of each of the elements of the system"[83] and to "understand internal technical communities/subcultures better."[84] This also meets Drucker's recommendation of requiring "extensive cross-disciplinary experience, from a systems perspective" in the development of a strategic leader.[85]

Garrison Health Services Unit. Normally, at the start of their career, CFHS personnel must consolidate their professional skills and their understanding of the CFHS garrison clinic as an operational readiness enabler for CF personnel in the more predictable in-garrison environment. Thus, their professional skills will be instinctive at the point they move on to a CFHS field unit to apply them in the less-predictable operational environment. This garrison experience and experience in a health services field unit is the entry-level aspect of the required "tactical- and operational-level expertise" discussed by interview participants, and it will serve to both hone their technical skill sets and broaden their perspective of the CF.[86]

Health Services Field Unit. Given the primacy of operations in the CF, experience in a health services field unit is another key foundational experience, following experience in a garrison health services unit, to prepare CFHS leaders both for deployment and for future leadership positions. It is here that they will also undertake the training to prepare for deployed operations, and be immersed in the culture of the line operational units served by the CFHS.

Operational Deployment. Interview participants saw "deployments … [as] a necessary foundation for strategic leadership,"[87] which is further supported by Smith's "broad and deep operational experience" requirement for strategic leaders.[88] The emphasis on this element is also in keeping with McGuire's interviews with US General Officers, who rated operational assignments as having been the most important developmental experiences in their careers.[89] Be it domestic or foreign, a deployment develops officers by allowing them to experience first hand the raison d'être for the CFHS: support to deployed operations.

Subunit, Unit and Group Command. There was a strong sense amongst interview participants of the essential nature of command as a requisite developmental element for strategic leaders as a way to give them credibility both within the CFHS and in the larger CF because "command is the 'currency' that all [CF] environments accept at par."[90] This is further supported by Johnson, who notes that "command is pre-eminent in the hierarchy of importance of assignments."[91] Command is so highly valued as a learning and performance experience within the military community because it entails both the ultimate authority and the ultimate accountability for the accomplishment of one's mission and for the well-being of the personnel under one's command. Command assignments are normally undertaken at progressively increasing levels of complexity throughout a career, with escalating levels of magnitude of the scale, scope and timespan of command duties.[92]

Headquarters Employment. The notion that potential CFHS strategic leaders should have experience in national-level headquarters was strongly supported by interview participants and by a former CDS, who stated that a lack of experience at NDHQ led to an unnecessarily steep learning curve later in his career that he felt initially diminished his performance as a strategic leader.[93] The common feeling among them was that, starting in DP 3A, "the experience of posting within National Defence Headquarters (NDHQ) is essential in developing strategic leaders,"[94] and that these experiences should include "key staff positions at the operational or strategic level."[95]

Other Government Departments (OGD) and Allied Employment. Besides proficiency in working within their own environment, strategic military leaders "must be able to effectively interface with government" and must be "able to navigate outside one's own culture, both internationally and domestically."[96] Interview participants emphasized the value of exchange postings with Allied militaries and with OGDs, national Canadian institutions and industry in order to broaden the perspective of future strategic leaders. It was also noted that such OGD experiences were important to develop a strategic-level understanding of government policies and practices.[97] They also described how other nations' militaries use a wide variety of exchanges as an organizational development initiative, whereby as a learning organization, these militaries maintain an external awareness by participating in exchange programs to "develop experiences and bring back insights."[98] This is in keeping with Fulkerson's recommendations for the necessary experiential elements for global leaders, which include experiences in "foreign" environments to develop deep awareness of other cultures.[99] It is these sorts of experiences that will give strategic CFHS leaders the cultural adaptability, cross-cultural savvy and global awareness to function effectively in the JIMP environment at the strategic level.[100]

To ensure equality of access to such exchange opportunities for CFHS officers, appropriate officers should be selected through the CFHS succession planning process to which all CFHS officers have equal access through their achievements and demonstrated potential.

Out-of-Health-Services CF Employment. In addition to exchanges with OGDs and Allied militaries, "out of trade" experiences were well supported as avenues of development for strategic leaders, and it was recommended that the CFHS "plan beyond the health services world" to effect this development.[101] Indeed, as the function of the CFHS is to support CF line organizations in their operational role, it would behoove the CFHS to work integrally in as many operational environments as possible. This experience would help the CFHS to be capable of effectively predicting and meeting the line organizations' health care needs in a systematic manner that is consonant with their respective organizational practices. Moreover, this experience would also serve to facilitate the strategic leader activity of further extending CFHS's influence beyond the HS organization.[102]

ORGANIZATIONAL IMPLEMENTATION OF THE STUDY'S RECOMMENDATIONS

> There is nothing more difficult to take in hand, more perilous to conduct, or more uncertain in its success, than to take the lead in the introduction of a new order of things. Because the innovator has for enemies all those who have done well under the old conditions, and lukewarm defenders in those who may do well under the new.[103]
>
>   Machiavelli, 1515

The CFHS needs a sustainable strategic leadership capacity to ensure that it is successful in adapting to the changing security environment. This capacity must be provided by a standardized and transparent process, something the HS community has lacked in the past. The CFHS Leader Development Framework presented here represents a further step in the definition of the processes currently required to develop future strategic-level CFHS leaders. Nevertheless, the Framework, by itself, will not resolve all the issues involved in the development of future strategic-level CFHS leaders. For example, Smith described the significant resource commitment involved in the PME process for US Air Force officers, including the assumption that strategic leader development would take place over the span of a 35-year career.[104] The CFHS dynamic has three further overlays. Firstly, given the change in generational demographics and its associated dynamics in Western militaries,[105] the demographic group currently being considered as part of the CFHS succession planning process will not likely be planning on a 35-year career; indeed, given recent changes to the CF terms of service, even career-minded CFHS officers in this demographic will probably tend to be seeking a 25-year career. Secondly, the CFHS has a large demographic of officers in clinical occupations which demand a further specific set of regulated qualifications and credentials, and which require, therefore, significant investment of resources, energy and expertise to initially gain and subsequently maintain these qualifications. Thirdly, unlike line officer occupations whose function is essentially to train for deployment and to deploy, with interspersed career development postings in staff and training positions, the CFHS has a further real-time activity which is the key element of its mission: the provision of health care to enable the operational readiness of the CF.

Thus, if the CFHS Executive chooses to accept a framework similar to the one presented here to guide the development future strategic-level CFHS leaders, given the commitment of resources that it would entail, some choices will have to be made. Firstly, the human resource (HR) and financial resources required for each potential strategic-leader aspirant would have to be calculated, and sought through the CF chain of command. This step would likely entail an increase in financial resources for training costs, and an increase in personnel establishment to reflect the increased training/education commitment and the commitment to increase the number of personnel serving outside of the CFHS for experiential purposes. Next, the CFHS leadership would need to continue to focus on the succession planning process, such that scarce resources are devoted to a limited number of candidates who truly reflect the possession of, or the ready capability of acquiring, the required competencies for strategic CFHS leadership. Finally, once the resource and time commitments have been calculated and considered in the light of resource and time requirements for the development and maintenance of clinical credentials, as well as the ongoing health care provision capacity requirements of the CFHS, the CFHS Executive would have to determine how CFHS officers in clinical occupations, having been identified through the succession planning process, could undertake the appropriate development activities in preparation for strategic leadership positions in the CFHS.

While some might think that CFHS strategic leader development is too costly in terms of resources, comparing it to strategic leader development for CF pilots may put it in context. For example, CF-18 pilots are arguably more expensive to train and keep current with regard to their complex professional and technical skills than CFHS clinicians. High potential officers in this military occupation tend to alternate between flying positions and staff/training/exchange positions, progressing from an "Element Leader" flying position in DP 2, to a "Flight Commander" flying position in DP 3A, to a "Squadron CO" flying position in DP 3B, to a "Wing Commander" partial flying position in DP 4. To do so, they have successfully (and evidently seamlessly) renewed their flight credentials on each occasion, and managed to undertake the full spectrum of CF leader development in the process. Moreover, members of this occupation have also gone on to successfully compete, at various times, for a great number of the strategic-level positions in NDHQ, including CDS.

CONCLUSION

Current CFHS leaders now function in a significantly more complex leadership environment than ever before, where legacy skill sets are no longer sufficient. This research project considered the question of how the CFHS could build a sustainable strategic leadership capacity that would meet the challenges of the future leadership environment, recognizing that strategic leader development is a key requirement for sustainability of an organization that has undergone significant internal transformational change in recent years involving its structure, culture and roles. The answer to this question was sought through a selective overview of the associated literature and a rigorous series of iterative qualitative research processes involving both internal and external stakeholders.

Three overarching themes emerged from the research data. The first was that CFHS colonels should have strategic-level competencies in common with other CF colonels; the second was that CFHS colonels must have an in-depth understanding of CF operations; and the third was that military, not civilian corporate, leader development models should be emphasized in CFHS strategic leader development. These data, refined through further qualitative research approaches, led to the development of a CFHS Leader Development Framework. This Framework addresses the "dual competencies," comprising both general CF knowledge and HS professional knowledge, required of CFHS officers. Elements in the Framework are grouped within the overarching domains of Military Training and Education, HS Professional Knowledge, and Experience, with the expressed component elements representing activities in the context of the CF officer development periods.

Implementation of the CFHS Leader Development Framework will likely be complicated by three key internal factors extant in the CFHS. First, the oft-chosen abbreviated career paths of our current DP3 demographic will likely require the concentration of development elements into a shorter career time span. Second, the requirement for the parallel and simultaneous achievement and maintenance of civilian health care credentials by CFHS personnel will add further organizational time pressures to the leader development process. And, finally, the requirement for the CFHS to have its personnel undertake the elements of a generic CF officer career path while ensuring the accomplishment of the tangible deliverables of the CFHS' organizational mission, namely the operational readiness of the CF population, will require the support by the CF leadership for a fundamental reassessment of CFHS human resource models.

While the cost of developing a sustainable strategic leadership capacity for the CFHS may be high, this cost is exceeded only by the cost of not developing this capacity to meet the needs of the CF.

NOTES

1   John de Chastelain, "A Personal Perspective on Command," in Bernd Horn and Stephen Harris, eds., *Warrior Chiefs: Perspectives On Senior Canadian Military Leaders* (Toronto: Dundurn Press, 2001), 352.

2   See J.C. Taylor, "CFHS Heal Thyself: Developing Strategic Health Services Leaders for the Modern Milieu," unpublished Master's thesis, Royal Roads University, 2005 for details.

3   US Army, *Army Leadership: Be-Know-Do*, Field Manual 22-100 (Washington, DC: US Department of the Army, 1999), p. 7-1.

4   Interviews conducted as part of research for J.C. Taylor, "CFHS Heal Thyself: Developing Strategic Health Services Leaders for the Modern Milieu," [hereafter "Interviews"], 6.

5   "Interviews," 7.

6   Ibid.

7   "Interviews," 8.

8   "Interviews," 7.

9   "Interviews," 5.

10   "Interviews," 6.

11   See G.E. Sharpe and Allan English, *Principles for Change in the Post-Cold War Command and Control of the Canadian Forces* (Kingston, ON: Canadian Forces Leadership Institute, 2002) for details.

12   "Interviews," 6.

13   "Interviews," 3.

14   "Interviews," 6. This comment is further supported by James M. Smith, "Expeditionary Leaders, CINCs and Chairmen: Shaping Air Force Officers for Leadership Roles in the Twenty-First Century, *Aerospace Power Journal* 14, no. 4 (Winter 2000), 30-44; and Mark A. McGuire, "Senior Officers and Strategic Leader Development," *Joint Force Quarterly* no. 29, (Autumn-Winter 2001/2002), 91-6.

15   "Interviews," 6. The Framework is further supported by recommendations to employ an adult education model in R.A. Chilcoat, *Strategic Art: The New Discipline for 21st Century Leaders* (Carlisle Barracks,
PA: US Army War College Paper, 1995); and by the American Productivity and Quality Center (APQC)
best practices report, APQC, *Leadership Development: Building Executive Talent* (Houston, TX: APQC,
1999). The distinction between education and training is discussed in the APQC report and in depth by
S. Lester, "Overcoming the Education-Training Divide: The Case of Professional Development," *Redland
Papers* (Autumn 1996), 1-8, available at http://www.devmts.demon.co.uk/divide.htm, accessed 18
January 2005; and US Air Force, *Leadership and Force Development*, Air Force Doctrine Document 1-1
(Washington, DC: US Department of the Air Force, 2004).

16   "Interviews," 5.

17   "Interviews," 1.

18   "Interviews," 3.

19   "Interviews," 7.

20   The DPs are roughly equivalent to rank as follows: DP 1 – Lieutenant, DP 2- Captain, DP 3A -
Major, DP 3B- Lieutenant-Colonel, and DP 4 - Colonel and General/Flag Officer.

21   M.A. Dalton and C.T. Ernst, "Developing Leaders for Global Roles," in C.D. McCauley and E. van
Velsor, eds., *The Center for Creative Leadership Handbook of Leadership Development* (San Francisco:
Jossey-Bass 2004), 366.

22   Kenneth H. Pritchard, "Competency-based Leadership for the 21st Century," *Military Review* 79,
no. 3 (May-June1999), 23.

23   "Interviews," 1.

24   "Interviews," 3.

25   Michael Flowers, "Improving Strategic Leadership," *Military Review* 84, no. 2 (March-
April 2004), 40-6.

26   US Chairman of the Joint Chiefs of Staff (CJCS), "CJCS Instruction 1800.01A: Officer Professional
Military Education Policy, dated1 December 2000, p. A-B-1, available at http://www.nwc.navy.mil/aca-
demics/images/1800_01a.pdf, accessed 20 August 2004.

27   W. Michael Guillot, "Strategic Leadership: Defining the Challenge," *Air and Space Power Journal* 17,
no. 4 (Winter 2003), 73.

28   See APQC, *Leadership Development: Building Executive Talent*.

29   Ibid., 48.

30   Ibid., 43, 51, 69. Smith, in "Expeditionary Leaders, CINCs and Chairmen," gave an overview of the
magnitude of the resources required to develop each military leader to the strategic level.

31   Canada, Department of National Defence (DND), *Leadership in the Canadian Forces: Conceptual
Foundations* (Kingston, ON: Canadian Defence Academy, 2005), 125.

32   See APQC, *Leadership Development: Building Executive Talent*.

33   "Interviews," 5.

34   DND, Defence Administrative Order and Directive (DAOD) 5031-7, "Initial Baccalaureate
Degree Programme," dated 13 Sep 2000, available at http://www.smafinsm.forces.gc.ca/admfincs/ sub-
jects/daod/5031/intro_e.asp

35   L. Wong, et al., *Strategic Leadership Competencies* (Carlisle Barracks, PA: US Army War College
Paper, 2003).

36   J.R. Fulkerson, "Growing Global Executives," in R. Silzer, ed., *The 21st Century Executive* (San
Francisco: Jossey-Bass, 2002), 315.

37   "Interviews," 5.

38   "Interviews," 1. See Wong, et al., *Strategic Leadership Competencies* for a discussion of the
tactical/technical foundation for strategic leadership competencies.

39   "Interviews," 1.

40   S. Paquet, et al., "Strategic Leadership Competencies in the Canadian Forces," unpublished paper

written for the Canadian Forces Leadership Institute (2003). Citation from Fulkerson, "Growing Global Executives," 315.

41   "Interviews," 7.

42   R.R. Magee, *Strategic Leadership Primer* (Carlisle Barracks, PA: US Army War College Paper, 1998).

43   McGuire, "Senior Officers and Strategic Leader Development," 91-6.

44   Wong, et al., *Strategic Leadership Competencies*.

45   "Interviews," 1. See for example S. J. Zaccaro, "Social Complexity and the Competencies Required for Effective Military Leadership," in J. G. Hunt, et al., eds. *Out-of-the-box Leadership: Transforming the Twenty-first-century Army and other Top-performing Organizations* (Stamford, CT: JAI Press, Inc., 1999), 131-151; Smith, "Expeditionary Leaders, CINCs and Chairmen"; Wong, et al., *Strategic Leadership Competencies*; and Pritchard, "Competency-based Leadership for the 21ˢᵗ Century."

46   "Interviews," 4.

47   "Interviews," 2.

48   "Interviews," 8.

49   "Interviews," 5.

50   This view is supported by Wong, et al., *Strategic Leadership Competencies*.

51   Smith, "Expeditionary Leaders, CINCs and Chairmen."

52   "Interviews," 2, 3. These views were supported by Wong, et al., *Strategic Leadership Competencies*; and J.A. Conger, "The Brave New World of Leadership Training, *Organizational Dynamics* 21, no. 3, (1993), 46-58.

53   Chilcoat, *Strategic Art*, 14.

54   Magee, *Strategic Leadership Primer*, 42.

55   Chilcoat, *Strategic Art*, 5.

56   Wong, et al., *Strategic Leadership Competencies*; Flowers, "Improving Strategic Leadership"; J. Horey, et al., *Competency Based Future Leadership Requirements* (Alexandria, VA: US Army Research Institute. 2004); and Smith, "Expeditionary Leaders, CINCs and Chairmen."

57   "Interviews," 2.

58   Wong, et al., *Strategic Leadership Competencies*.

59   McGuire, "Senior Officers and Strategic Leader Development," 91-6.

60   "Interviews," 7.

61   DND, *Leadership in the Canadian Forces: Doctrine* (Kingston, ON: Canadian Defence Academy, 2005).

62   Horey, et al., *Competency Based Future Leadership Requirements*, 42.

63   DND, *Leadership in the Canadian Forces: Conceptual Foundations*.

64   "Interviews," 3.

65   DND, *Leadership in the Canadian Forces: Conceptual Foundations*.

66   APQC, *Leadership Development: Building Executive Talent*; and D.V. Day and S.M. Halpin, Leadership Development: A Review of Industry Best Practices (Alexandria, VA: US Army Research Institute, 2001).

67   "Interviews," 7.

68   Conference Board, *The Business Value of Leadership Development* (New York: The Conference Board, Inc., 2005), 366.

69   US Army Medical Department, Office of Medical History, "The Surgeons-General of the US Army and their Predecessors," available at http://history.amedd.army.mil. Accessed 10 June 2005.

70   These views are supported by Magee, *Strategic Leadership Primer*; Wong, et al., *Strategic Leadership Competencies*; and Horey, et al., *Competency Based Future Leadership Requirements*.

71   Wong, et al., *Strategic Leadership Competencies*.

72   Chilcoat, *Strategic Art*,14.

73   This point is supported by Magee, *Strategic Leadership Primer*.

74   Joint Medical Executive Skills Institute, *Joint Medical Executive Skills Program Core Curriculum* (San

Antonio, TX: Joint Medical Executive Skills Institute, 2004)

75   APQC, *Leadership Development: Building Executive Talent*, 65.

76   "Interviews," 7.

77   "Interviews," 6.

78   "Interviews," 5.

79   "Interviews," 1.

80   These views are supported by Magee, *Strategic Leadership Primer*; Horey, et al., *Competency Based Future Leadership Requirements*; and Chilcoat, *Strategic Art*, 14.

81   Flowers, "Improving Strategic Leadership."

82   "Interviews," 2.

83   "Interviews," 6.

84   "Interviews," 8.

85   P.F. Drucker, *The Executive in Action: Three Classic Works on Management* (New York: HarperCollins, 1996), 271.

86   "Interviews," 5.

87   "Interviews," 7.

88   Smith, "Expeditionary Leaders, CINCs and Chairmen," 32.

89   McGuire, "Senior Officers and Strategic Leader Development," 91-6.

90   "Interviews," 8.

91   D.E. Johnson, *Preparing Potential Senior Army Leaders for the Future* (Santa Monica, CA: RAND Arroyo Center, 2002), 23.

92   T.O. Jacobs and Elliot Jaques, "Executive Leadership," in R. Gal. and D. Mangelsdorff, eds., *Handbook of Military Psychology* (West Sussex, UK: Wiley, 1991), 75-94.

93   de Chastelain, "A Personal Perspective on Command," 353.

94   "Interviews," 4.

95   "Interviews," 7.

96   "Interviews," 4.

97   This point is supported by Guillot, "Strategic Leadership: Defining the Challenge."

98   "Interviews," 4.

99   Fulkerson, "Growing Global Executives." Similar recommendations were expressed in the US National Aeronautics and Space Administration's (NASA) leadership development model – NASA, "Leadership Development Model," available at http://leadership.nasa.gov/nasa/lmd/Model/SixNav/SixNav_IE.asp, accessed 18 July 2004.

100   These characteristics were supported by Conference Board, *The Business Value of Leadership Development*; Wong, et al., *Strategic Leadership Competencies*; Conger, "The Brave New World of Leadership Training"; and Flowers, "Improving Strategic Leadership."

101   "Interviews," 7.

102   Horey, et al., *Competency Based Future Leadership Requirements*.

103   N. Machiavelli, *The Prince*, W.K. Marriott, trans., (Adelaide, Australia: University of Adelaide Library, Electronic Texts Collection, 2004, originally published 1515), available at http://etext.library.adelaide.edu.au/m/machiavelli/niccolo/m149p/ accessed 15 March 2005, Chapter 6, np.

104   Smith, "Expeditionary Leaders, CINCs and Chairmen."

105   As described in Wong, et al., *Strategic Leadership Competencies*.

CONCLUSION

Allan English and Colonel James C. Taylor

The purpose of this book was to contribute to the growing literature on how Health Service Support (HSS) can be transformed to meet the challenges of the current and future security environments. In so doing, it also aimed to complement the two previous books in this series, *The Operational Art: Canadian Perspectives – Context and Concepts* and *The Operational Art: Canadian Perspectives – Leadership and Command*. All three books in the series share the premise that there are unique Canadian approaches to operational art based on our national and military culture and historical experience. We believe that Canadian military professionals should become familiar with these approaches so that the practice of their profession will be based on sound theory as well as their personal experience.

The chapters in this volume are representative of some of Canada's contributions to the ongoing doctrinal discussion among North Atlantic Treaty Organization (NATO) nations regarding the evolution of HSS in the new security environment, which itself is evolving and has been described by terms like "Joint, Interagency, Multinational, and Public" (JIMP), "3D" (defence, diplomacy and development), and "integrated." The inclusion of this volume within the Canadian Defence Academy's operational art series indicates that the Canadian Forces (CF), like its NATO partners, sees HSS as an integral element of operational planning, and that the neglect of HSS in the operational planning process puts campaigns and those who execute them in grave peril.

In order to ensure that campaigns achieve their objectives, practitioners of the operational art must be cognizant of, and include in their plans, HSS factors. For "operators" this means that they must have a solid understanding of the doctrine and roles of their HSS elements. For HSS personnel this means that, as "dual professionals," they must master the "common body of knowledge" of the profession of arms in Canada as well as their civilian professional body of knowledge. For selected senior HSS personnel, this military professional body of knowledge includes aspects of the operational art so that they can contribute effectively to the planning and execution of campaigns. It also includes mastering strategic concepts so that HSS senior leaders can ensure that HSS continues to be responsive to the needs of its clients in the new security environment. Important enablers of these outcomes are new concepts and doctrine on support to joint and combined operations, including HSS concepts, doctrine, and policies in a Canadian context. Therefore, this book was commissioned by the Commander Canadian Forces Health Services (CFHS) Group to provide a contribution to the debate on these issues.

The first two chapters in this volume, drawing on historical and current examples, depicted how military operations might be conducted in the new security environment, and suggested ways that would make HSS more responsive to the needs of the CF in the post-Cold War world. Both chapters shared the view that changes in society, demographics, technology, and health care practice will significantly impact how health care services are provided in the future, as both health care providers' and their clients' expectations of what constitutes appropriate health care evolve. These trends, it was concluded, will also impact the CF; therefore, the CF must anticipate these changes and be prepared to deal with them effectively. In order to do so, the authors of the first two chapters argued that CF leaders at all levels must have the knowledge and the will to implement appropriate measures. Unfortunately for the CF, this has not always been the case in the past. To rectify this shortcoming, the authors indicated that formal educational requirements that are progressive and appropriate to leaders' levels of responsibility would be one way to address the challenges of providing appropriate HSS in the future. Education, however, must be complemented by an understanding by all CF leaders, both "operators" and specialists, of their roles in providing effective health care to members of the CF.

The next four chapters challenged, modified, and built on the views of military operations in the new security environment presented in the first two chapters. The authors of these four chapters debated the requirements for a deployable HSS capability that is valid across all CF force planning scenarios, that is benchmarked to a Canadian civilian level of care, and that is interoperable with our principal allies. The authors of the first three chapters in this part of the book all agreed that, due to limitations in aeromedical evacuation, some form of robust forward surgical and evacuation capability would be required in the foreseeable future. While differing in details, these authors agreed that the current CF field ambulance capabilities and doctrine will need to be modified if HSS is to be able to adequately support CF units in the future battlespace. Those planning these modifications will need to balance the competing demands of such factors as mobility and definitive treatment, the location of surgical capabilities, and the proper skill set of medical personnel in support of future operations. The final chapter in this part addressed dental aspects of HSS in the future battlespace, and concluded that, as with other HSS capabilities, dental health services support to operations should be organized around modular, building block capabilities that are readily deployable, modern, and interoperable with our allies. Since all the authors in this part concluded that changes in equipment, organization and doctrine are required to assure effective HSS in the new security environment, it is clear that how these changes should be achieved is a fertile field for future research and debate.

The final two chapters of the book provided some perspectives on this debate by discussing issues that impact on how the CF can best address required changes in equipment, organization and doctrine, especially those changes related to HSS, as transformation proceeds apace. In the penultimate chapter, the Canadian Navy's multipurpose Joint Support Ship (JSS) was presented as a case study in how HSS considerations could affect operational planning. The author argued that JSS capabilities may be degraded if the competing priorities of multi-tasking are not considered in the planning process, as committing the JSS to one type of major task may seriously affect its ability to carry out another major task, or tasks, simultaneously. This problem could be addressed in CF joint doctrine, but to date, none has been produced to tackle this issue. The author of the last chapter examined how the senior leadership of the CFHS can best be prepared to deal with future challenges. He argued that if CF HSS is to be effective in the new, more complex, leadership environment of today and tomorrow, the CFHS must have a sustainable strategic leadership development process that is both standardized and transparent. A CFHS Leader Development Framework, based on military leader development models, was proposed by the author to attempt to resolve the "dual competencies" and "dual professionals" conundrum faced by HSS personnel. The Framework proposed ways of solving this so that CFHS strategic leaders would have strategic-level competencies in common with their peers as well as an in-depth understanding of CF operations. While there would be substantial costs to adopting the approach advocated here, the author pointed out that the cost of not developing a sustainable strategic leadership capacity for the CFHS would be greater.

The CF faces many challenges in the new security environment. Among these challenges is the effective planning and execution of campaigns that include increasingly "integrated" teams. To be successful in this new environment, practitioners of the operational art will need to master many skills. Among these skills is the ability to understand how support factors, and HSS in particular, affect operational-level activities. Too often in the past HSS has been relegated to the support "afterthought" part of the campaign planning process, with predictably serious negative effects on the campaign. To avoid these problems in the future, operational-level commanders, their staffs, and their HSS advisors will need to understand the critical role that HSS plays in the planning and execution of campaigns and will also need to be able to apply that understanding appropriately. However, if commanders, staff officers and specialist advisors are to acquire the necessary skills in the application of the operational art, relevant theory, experience, and doctrine must be readily available to them. Furthermore, HSS strategic leaders must be aware of how HSS should evolve to support future campaigns and cause it to transform in ways that ensure its continued effectiveness. The contributions here are offered as part of these processes.

CONTRIBUTORS

COLONEL JEAN-ROBERT BERNIER, CD, BA (Hons), MD, MPH, DEH, is Director Force Health Protection for the Canadian Forces. A graduate of the Royal Military College of Canada, he served as an infantry officer (Princess Patricia's Canadian Light Infantry) in regimental, instructional, and brigade operations staff positions prior to training as a physician. He served in medical officer appointments in Canada and Germany before completing post-graduate training in public health, environmental health, medical intelligence, intelligence analysis, and chemical/biological/radiological (CBR) casualty management at US Defence Department universities and institutions. He subsequently served as an intelligence analyst with the US Defence Intelligence Agency, directed military operational medicine and occupational/environmental health for the Canadian Forces, and was chair or vice-chair of several allied medical CBR and intelligence committees prior to assuming his current appointment. He is a graduate of the Land Force Command and Staff College and the Advanced Military Studies Course and is an elected member of Delta Omega, the US public health honour society.

ALLAN ENGLISH, CD, BA (Hons), MA, PhD, was the lead academic for the Advanced Military Studies Course from its inception in 1998 to 2004 and he was Co-chair of the Aerospace Studies Department from 2001 to 2005 at the Canadian Forces College. He is an Adjunct Associate Professor of History at Queen's University where he teaches a graduate course in Canadian military history. His book *Understanding Military Culture: A Canadian Perspective* (2004) is published by McGill-Queen's University Press. He co-edited *The Operational Art: Canadian Perspectives – Context and Concepts* (2005) and edited *The Operational Art: Canadian Perspectives – Leadership and Command* (2006), both published by the Canadian Defence Academy Press.

LIEUTENANT-COLONEL C.L. MITCHELL, CD, BA, MA, is a Health Services Operations officer who has served in a number of field and staff positions throughout her career. She was promoted to the rank of Lieutenant-Colonel in August 2002. From 2002-2005, she commanded 1 Canadian Field Hospital, CFB Petawawa. She is a graduate of the Land Forces Command and Staff Course, held at Kingston, and the Advanced

Military Studies Course, held at Canadian Forces College Toronto. She holds a BA in psychology and a MA in leadership and training. She is currently the Chief of Staff, 1 Health Services Group Headquarters located in Garrison Edmonton.

MAJOR (RETIRED) STEPHEN MOLYNEAUX, CD, BSc, DDS, was a Dental Officer in the Canadian Forces. He joined the CF as a dental student in 1986 and graduated from the University of Western Ontario with a DDS. degree in 1990. He has served as a Dental Officer at CFB Kingston, the Royal Military College of Canada, and the NATO Airbase at Geilenkirchen. He was Dental Platoon Commander at 1 Field Ambulance in Edmonton and Staff Officer for Dental Operations at the Directorate of Dental Services in Ottawa. He is a graduate of Command and Staff Course 31, Canadian Forces College. Major Molyneaux retired from the position of Detachment Commander at 1 Dental Unit Detachment Borden.

COMMANDER REBECCA PATTERSON, CD, BSN, CHE, is a Health Services Operations (HSO) officer who has held unit command positions at the Canadian Forces Medical Services School, CFB Borden and the Canadian Forces Health Services Centre (Atlantic), Halifax. A former critical care Nursing Officer, she served as a member of 1 Canadian Field Hospital during *Operation Scalpel* (Gulf and Kuwait Conflict 1991) and as a member of the Advanced Surgical Team supporting the Airborne Regiment during *Operation Deliverance* (Somalia 1993). In 1997, she transferred to HSO and has been an active participant in the transformation of the CF Health Services. She holds a Bachelor of Science Nursing/ Primary Health Care Nurse Practitioner certificate, is a Certified Health Services Executive and is a graduate of the Advanced Military Studies Course. She is currently posted to second language training at CFB Shearwater.

COLONEL (RETIRED) DAVID SALISBURY, CD, MD, MHSc, is the Medical Officer of Health for the City of Ottawa and a Senior Consultant in Aviation Medicine to Transport Canada's Civil Aviation Medicine Branch. He graduated from Queen's University Medical School at Kingston in 1978 and was a flight surgeon in the Canadian Forces for almost thirty years retiring at the rank of Colonel. He has a Masters degree in Occupational Health from the University of British Columbia and graduated from the US Air Force Residency in Aerospace Medicine course in 1988. During his military aviation medicine career he was Head of Central Medical Board, Medical Advisor to the Chief of the Air Staff and Commanding Officer of the Canadian Forces Environmental Medicine Establishment better known as DCIEM. He has numerous publications in aviation medicine, occupational medicine, epidemiology and public health. He has been the President of the International Military Flight Surgeon Pilots Association, the Canadian Aerospace Medicine and Aeromedical Transport Association and is a Fellow of the Aerospace Medical Association. He is an active pilot and is Board Certified in Aerospace Medicine as well as being a Fellow of the Royal College of Physicians and Surgeons of Canada in Community Medicine.

COLONEL JAMES C. TAYLOR, CD, BSc, DMD, MA, Cert Prostho, is a Dental Specialist Officer who currently commands 1 Dental Unit, which comprises all Canadian Forces garrison Dental capability in Canada and Europe. Having undertaken both his undergraduate and dental school studies at the University of British Columbia in Vancouver, he served in a series of appointments as a line Dental Officer, Ship's Dental Officer, Platoon Commander and Detachment Commander. He then served in a series of staff appointments in Canadian Forces Health Services Group Headquarters, including G3 Dental (Dental Operations & Plans), Director Dental Services 3 (Dental Operations, Training & Recruiting) and G3 (Health Services Operations). He completed his clinical post-graduate training in Prosthodontics at Walter Reed Army Medical Center in Washington, DC, his Master of Arts degree at Royal Roads University in Victoria, BC, and the Advanced Military Studies Course 5 at Canadian Forces College. Along with his command position, he maintains a part-time clinical Prosthodontic practice at the National Defence Medical Centre in Ottawa.

In the civilian professional community, Colonel Taylor is an Assistant Professor in the Division of Prosthodontics at the Dalhousie University Faculty of Dentistry and a Member of both the Faculty of Graduate Studies and the Dalhousie Institute for Research in Materials. He is also a Past President of the Association of Prosthodontists of Canada and is currently the Chair of the Academy of Osseointegration Council on Research, and the national representative for Prosthodontics on the Canadian Dental Association's (CDA's) Committee on Specialty Affairs. Col Taylor serves as a reviewer and/or member of the Editorial Board for six clinical journals internationally, and received the 2001 award for Best Article in the International Journal of Oral and Maxillofacial Implants. He holds Membership in the Association of Prosthodontists of Canada, the American College of Prosthodontists, and the International College of Prosthodontists, and holds Fellowship in the Academy of Prosthodontics, the Academy of Osseointegration, the Academy of Dentistry International, the International College of Dentists, and the Inter-University Seminar on Armed Forces and Society. He was a 2004 recipient of the CDA Award of Merit, and a 2006 recipient of the CDA Certificate of Merit.

LIEUTENANT-COLONEL DAVID R. WEGER, CD, BA, MPH, CHE, is a Health Services Operations officer with 25 years service in the CF. He has commanded at the unit level, deployed on both domestic and expeditionary operations, and held staff appointments in tactical, operational and strategic level headquarters. He is a graduate of the Canadian Forces Staff School, the Canadian Land Force Command and Staff College, and the Advanced Military Studies Course. He holds a BA (Military and Strategic Studies) from Royal Roads Military College and a Master of Public Health (Health Policy and Management) from the University of Alberta. Lieutenant-Colonel Weger is currently serving as G5/G7 Plans, Training and Doctrine with the Canadian Forces Medical Group Headquarters in Ottawa. In this capacity he is responsible for strategic level health service support operational planning, collective training, doctrine development, and NATO and ABCA analysis.

INDEX